LEWY WHO?

By: *JJ Johnstone*

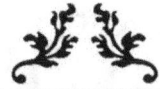

All rights reserved. The use of any part of this publication reproduced, transmitted in any form or by any means, electronic, mechanical, photocopying, or otherwise, or stored in a retrieval system, without the prior written consent of the author, is an infringement of the copyright law.

Copyright: The SCOPYRIGHT.ca Team

Objective Concept LTD. Scopyright.ca register at RCS
PARIS B 500 790 910 – U.E.

Thank You to Andrew at:

Open Book Prints

When I first spoke to Andrew, he said "He likes to support a worthy cause."

He has been great. He has shown extreme kindness and generosity in getting this book printed and out to the public.

I am very grateful for all your help.

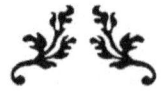

Open Book Prints

1380 Hopkins St.
Units 13 & 14
Whitby On.

905-706-3943

print@openbookprints.com

DISCLAIMER PAGE

This book does not endorse in any way any type of procedures for Parkinson's Disease or Lewy Body Disease.

The treatments that were pursued by John are strictly trial and error and knowing that everyone is different, and that people respond differently to medications and procedures, we are therefore not mentioning the names of drugs.

This book is written in hopes that it will help someone somewhere.

You are NOT ALONE.

There are caring individuals out there who are willing to help.

Proper diagnoses of many diseases are hard to get. Some diseases like Parkinson's disease and Lewy Body are given only after every other illness has been eliminated, and even then, it can still be a guess.

Also,

I do not accept any responsibility for any information about the Lewy Body, Dementia or Alzheimer's Disease. I have gotten information from many different sources.

There needs to be more research needs to be done in the area of Alzheimer's and different forms of Dementia.

The information that I inserted into the book was done so because I felt that it might be of interest to others and maybe answers some questions for people who have been wondering about their health or the health of a loved one. I am not a professional and have learned only by living with someone who has Lewy Body.

Always seek the help of professionals to give you a proper diagnosis.

ACKNOWLEDGEMENTS

I would like to Thank Adrian and Natalia Gallucci for donating some of their valuable time in helping to get this book together to make sure that it was ready for print and out on the market in time for the first anniversary of when the Lewy Body symptoms began. You are always there when needed. You're both Amazing people. We love you guys.

I would like to Thank John's Family Physician, Dr Jamie Read of The Trent Hills Family Health Team in Campbellford Ontario, he has been very instrumental in helping John. He has dedicated some of his off hours into researching this disease. He has treated John, as he does for all his patients, with dignity and respect. He is encouraging when needed and always available to listen and help where he can.

I want to Thank Dr Craig Cocek and his Amazing staff of Dr Cocek's Chiropractic Centre in Trenton for their fantastic support. Helping John stand a little taller and bend a bit better. Dr. Cocek's assistants are always providing a light-hearted atmosphere that is relaxing and enjoyable for John and many others.

I want to Thank Dr Sanjeev Sukumaran Au.D. and all the excellent staff from the Ear Company, in Peterborough. For being there any time John needed help and keeping his hearing aids serviced. Friendly smiles and words of encouragement mean a lot.

I want to give a big Thank You to family, friends and neighbours who are always there when needed and giving their loving support.

Last, but not least, I would like to Thank John. It has taken a lot of courage to allow a book to be written about his private life and what he faces each day with the Parkinson's and Lewy Body disease. He is sacrificing his privacy in hopes that it will help someone else out there. It takes a big man to give everything he has in hopes to help others. Thank You for your wonderful sense of humour.

This book is dedicated to all the people who live with Dementia and Alzheimer's.

Index

Chapter One:_____Pages 1 - 16

Chapter Two:_____Pages 17 - 38

Chapter Three:_____Pages 39 - 51

Chapter Four:_____Pages 52 - 64

Chapter Five:_____Pages 65 - 75

Chapter Six:_____Pages 76 - 93

Chapter Seven:_____Pages 94 - 108

Chapter Eight:_____Pages 109 - 122

Facts about Dementia:_____Pages 123 - 124

Facts about Parkinson's:_____Pages 125 - 126

Strange Facts:_____Pages 127 - 129

National Resources:_____Pages 130 - 136

Help Is Out There:_____Page 137

A Message for You:_____Pages 138 - 161

Notes:_____Pages 162 - 166

<u>CHAPTER ONE</u>

The store was full of Christmas shoppers and the rush of the holiday season had begun. It was only a couple of weeks before the big day, and it seemed like everyone from everywhere was trying hard to get the last minutes items. Christmas music sifted through the air putting people into the spirit of shopping. I noticed that a lady dressed in a red coat and hat hummed with the music as she picked up items off a shelf, looking at the price and then sitting it back down and then picking up something else. Decorations sparkled, and tinsel trees lined the counters, trying to get all shoppers into the mood to spend. Children ran through the store excitedly talking and laughing as they made their way to the toy department.

I was carrying a few items that I had picked up, and I turned around to look at John to find him standing leaning on a counter. His colour had changed from a healthy tan to a greyish tone. He seemed unsteady on his feet.

"Are you alright?" I asked with concern.

"I don't feel well. My legs are weak, and I feel shaky."

I looked around, and I could not see anywhere a place for him to sit down. I said, "Alright, let's take our time and try to get back to the car. Do you think that you can make it?"

He just shook his head yes and took a step away from the shelf. I could tell that he was feeling weak so I took hold of his arm and tried to steady him. I could see that he had to concentrate on each step that he made.

John's six foot two inch, two hundred pound frame was now leaning on me, and at this moment the difference in our sizes was very apparent, with me being only five feet two inches, and about a hundred pounds.

I could feel that he was becoming more unsteady with each step we took. I was having a hard time to bear his weight. I feared that I would let him fall and he would get hurt.

A few minutes later we were outside the store, and I was hoping that the fresh, crisp air would make him feel better, but it was plain to see that he continued to feel weak. His legs looked like they wanted to give out on him and I was concerned that he would fall on the pavement.

People were rushing by us going in and out of the store. The hectic scene on the sidewalk only seemed to make matters worse.

There was light snow that had started falling. A strong gust of wind whipped past us, and John looked as if a shiver had come over him.

"Take your time. There is no rush," I stated.

I tried to wrap the black canvas winter jacket; he was wearing, in front of him to work and keep out the wind so he wouldn't chill. He only had a thin plaid shirt on under his jacket, tucked into his blue jeans. I noticed that one of his steel-toed work boots, that he always insisted on wearing no matter what the occasion, was untied and I was afraid that with the way he was feeling, he could easily trip on the laces. I would have offered to bend down and tie them but I was afraid to let go of him, so I felt that we would take our chances and try to make it to the car.

I kept my eyes on his feet and watched every step that he took as he leaned on me
.

"There's our Buick Rendezvous right over there. Not much farther to go," I said as I tried to encourage him on. I felt that there was a couple of times that he just wanted to stop and standstill, but I was afraid that his legs were going to give out on him before getting to the car, so I tried to keep him moving.

Finally, we got to the vehicle, and I opened the passenger door and assisted him in. I handed him the seat belt, and then I opened the glove compartment and gave him a chocolate bar that I knew was in there. John held onto the bar, but it seemed he was in no shape to open it. So, I took it back from him and removed the wrapper and then gave it back to him, "Here take a few bites and see if that helps you feel any better."

He bit into the bar, and I closed the door. The wind blew my long blond hair into my face and eyes. I pushed the hair away, and then I pulled my black leather coat around me, to cut out the wind as I quickly made my way to the driver's door and then got into the car as well.

"Do you want to go to the Hospital?"

"No, I just want to go home."

I studied him for a moment. His blue eyes seemed sunken, and his brow was netted together with pain. His dark wavy hair looked messed up from the wind and his greying beard hide a lot of his pale skin on his face. He looked exhausted.

"Alright," I said as I started the car and drove out of the parking lot.

John had been diagnosed with Parkinson's disease two years ago. He had essential tremor for years, but in the past two years, it seemed to get a lot worse. He was living with daily pain, and we had gone to several Doctor's and had many tests done. Through the process of limitations of other diseases; finally, they diagnosed him with Parkinson's.

John didn't want to believe that he now had Parkinson's and he kept talking about how he was going to get better and someday the pain would be gone. Then he would be able to do all the things he wanted, but for now, they are on hold.

"No one knows for sure," he said. "One Doctor will say I have it and another Doctor will say he doesn't know for sure. So what am I to believe?"

"I guess it does not matter what label anyone wants to give it. What matters is how you feel, the quality of your life and has it changed your life any?" I responded.

He looked at me and said, "Well I don't have it as far as I'm concerned."

When I first met John in 2005, he was being treated then with Parkinson's medication for the Essential Tremor, but he hated the side effects that he was having and he decided to stop the medication. "I just never feel right when I am on this stuff," he had said to me. So with the help of his Doctor, he had gotten weaned off and just tried to ignore the tremor as much as possible. He adapted great for the most part. I was always amazed watching him build something as his hands would become steadier.

His love of tinkering and building things was on hold now. Everything he attempted to do was too painful and exhausting. Over the past couple of years, he had started some projects on the house, such as fixing up and redoing the floors and walls. John attempted giving the place a new facelift, but he was unable to complete any of them, due to the pain that he experienced. His family Doctor had tried him on many different types of pain medications but only to find that he had no tolerance to this type of medicines and would be sick to his stomach on top of everything else. I had even taken him to a pain clinic in Peterborough, but also that did not work for him. After about three times of being there and receiving pain medication into the spine, he finally gave it up as it did not work at all for him.

I had signed him up with a Doctor Craig Cocek a Chiropractor in Trenton, in the spring of 2017 to see if it would help John with any of his pain.

It seemed to help a bit with the way he stood and with his walking. He had started becoming bent over with the Parkinson's and the pain.

We were both very impressed with this Doctor as he had stated about how the brain works and that the brain and the spine working together can create many types of diseases if one or both stops working correctly. The Doctor also talked about his faith in God, and I thought that was a unique and very inspiring thing to tell his patients. It is rare to hear from professionals today, and I thought that was pretty refreshing. His office has kept close track of John's improvements as they do ex-rays and chat with us about the results and listen to any concerns we may have.

When we reached home, I helped John out of the car and into the house. I sat him down at the kitchen table and got him a coffee and a sandwich. He tried to get the hot liquid to his mouth but was having a hard time without spilling it. I could see the frustration on his face as the hot coffee splashed over his hands and onto the table.

"Don't worry," I said as I grabbed a piece of paper towel and wiped up the brown liquid.

Frustration showed on his face as he fought to get his sandwich to his mouth without having the bread fall apart. He held onto it so tightly that it started to disincarnate in his hands. The sandwich finally fell apart, and he tossed it onto the plate.

I went to the fridge and got out some cheese; I cut a piece and handed it to him. While he nibbled on it, I got some cookies and gave him one. I then took a bit of bread and threw it into the toaster.

In a couple of minutes I had buttered the toast and cut it up into small pieces, and he was able to handle that much better.

In about ten minutes, he started to look a bit better. He was now beginning to talk and pay attention to what I was saying and responding better than he had been before. His color had changed from the pale grey to a more golden colour.

"Feeling better?"

"Yes, I think I am starting to feel like my old self again. I'm not sure if that is a good thing or not," John responded with a smile.

I smiled back and said, "I am going outside to see how Adrian and Natalia and the kids are making out with the Christmas decorations."

My son Adrian, his wife Natalia and the twins aged six, Vince and Alyssa, were staying with us for a couple of weeks while they waited for a house they had purchased to be ready.

I found them outside where they worked hard at decorating the outside of the house. They had done a great job, with the deck of the house all decorated with tinsel and bows. They had set up a Christmas sleigh with reindeer that my neighbour and good friend had given me. Her father had made it in the 1950s for her family. As her children got, older no one seemed to want it so she asked if I would like to have it.

"I would be honoured to have it," I had responded.

It looked great at the front of the house. The twins were so excited about the job they had done and came running over to me to show me all of the work that they had helped to do.

"It looks fantastic out here. You have all worked hard on this. I appreciate it very much."

"No problem Grandma. We like doing it," responded Vince. His knitted hat was on sideways on his head with dark brown hair peeking out around the edges framing his red-cheeked face. His dark eyes sparkled with excitement.

"I helped too," said Alyssa as she walked towards me carrying a hand full of tinsel. Her long dark curls also framed a very red-cheeked face. Her dark brown eyes shone with delight as she held out the tinsel towards me, "I helped put this up on the railings of the deck."

As I got closer to Natalia, she smiled, and I noticed that her beautiful features where all red from the cold and her long dark hair was whipping in the wind that blew even stronger now. "We have almost finished, and then I think we will go inside and get a hot coffee to warm up. The sun is warm, but there is a chill in the air."

Adrian with a knitted hat on his head and gloves on his hands also smiled as he put the finishing touches on a railing on the stairs. The bows that hung on each side of the porch gave the front of the house a very festive look. His dark eyes also shone with excitement and his bronze face was now red as well with the cold, "Yes I could use a coffee."

"I just want to warn you that John is not feeling well," I said looking at them.

"What happened?" Adrian asked concerned.

"We were in the store, and he suddenly felt weak, and his tremor got terrible, his colour changed and we had to leave the store right away. I was afraid that he was going to fall. I was not sure if John was going to make it back to the car. I considered calling you guys to come and help me with him, but we made it."

"Oh no," said Natalia. "Is there anything that we can do?"

"Not really, I think we just need to act normal around him but still try and keep him calm and quiet if possible."

Just then, I saw my neighbour making her way up the sidewalk towards our house. She was talking to the kids as they surrounded her, giving her hugs and kisses. They had grown to love her and called her Grandma Bev.

I turned and walked down the deck toward her. I called out and said, "How are you?"

She laughed as she gave the kids hugs and then said, "I just wanted to come and say hello to everyone."

We all stood around talking for a couple of minutes, and then I noticed that John was making his way down the deck of the house. He walked as if his legs were weak. I hurried over to him and said, "Thought you would come out and get some fresh air?"

"Yes, I wanted to see the decorations and how everyone is making out."

"Look Grandpa we decorated the house for you," called out Alyssa.

"It looks like a nice job. Santa might find the house now that it is decorated," John smiled weakly.

Just then he swayed on his feet and looked like he was about to pass out. I grabbed him, and Bev reached out towards him as well.

"Lets' get you back inside," I said as I helped him turn around and then led him back towards the stairs."

"I'll talk to you guys later," called out Bev as she turned and walked back to her house.

We all made our way inside, and I got John to sit back down at the table. He looked exhausted at this point.

I looked at him and asked, "Would you like to go and lie down for a while?"

"No, I just want to sit still for a few minutes and then I will be fine."

The next morning, I was getting John dressed, and he sat down on the bed while I got his clothes ready to put on. He said to me, "Yesterday I had a strange occurrence."

"Oh, really what was that?"

"I was seeing people's faces distorted. They were cartoon-like. They would have an eye missing or an ear in the wrong place or a nose off to the side of a face. Everyone looked like cartoon characters."

I was shocked. I stayed quiet for a moment trying to digest what John had just said. Then I asked him, "Is this the first time it has ever happened?"

"No, I have never had that before."

"Why didn't you tell me yesterday?"

"I don't know. I'm telling you now," John responded.

I continued to feel shocked. I kept trying to process the information that John had just told me. I finished getting him dressed and then I asked him, "Do you have any distortions this morning?"

"No, I have not had any today."

A few minutes later we were back downstairs with Adrian and Natalia. They were in the kitchen discussing their move into the new house and when it might take place.

"We have heard that it might be another week before we can move into the house," Natalia said.

"That's alright. It is not an inconvenience for you to be here, the truth is we enjoy having you guys here, so don't rush on our part.," I responded smiling.

"We appreciate your help," they both responded at the same time.

"No worries," I smiled.

"John was telling me upstairs about something that happened to him yesterday.

It turns out that he started seeing people's faces distorted. He saw facial features such as an eye or nose in the wrong place."

"What were you are seeing John?" asked Adrian concerned.

"I was seeing people looking like cartoon characters. It looks bizarre to see someone with an eye in a forehead or a mouth where an eye should be."

Adrian and Natalia both had concerned looks on their faces as they listened to John explain the events the day before. We were all quiet while John continued to tell that everyone seemed distorted yesterday.

Adrian slowly asked, "How are you feeling now? Do you have any distortions today?"

"I feel better than I did yesterday and I have not had any distortions today."

Natalia grabbed her laptop computer and went onto Google. She tried to find what it might be. She finally came up with the name of a disease call Prosopometamorphopsia. This is a very rare visual perceptual distortion resulting in an altered perception of faces. Some people are describing the faces as being cartoon-like quality. "Wow! I have never heard of such a thing before."

"No I haven't, but it's good to put a name to it even if it is rare. At least we know kind of what is happening," I said as I looked over at John who was sitting in a chair looking confused about everything going on.

Adrian stood up to go and pour himself a coffee, and smiled at John and said, "Well John, would you like a coffee?"

"Sounds like a great idea," smiled John.

For the rest of the day, we were all on our guard and watching over John but yet not trying to make too much of a fuss. "We need to act naturally around him," I said.

"We agree, but it's hard not to worry about what might be going on with him," said Natalia.

"Well let's just do the same things we would have done if this was not happening as I believe that he would not want us to start treating him as if something was wrong," I smiled.

Later that day John and I sat in the kitchen, and I asked him, "Have you had any distortions today?"

"Only one and it was of someone on the TV."

Over the next few days, John started talking about having the distortions more and more. They had started with one or two a day and just seemed to get worse each day. They would last longer and became more frequent. I started keeping track on a calendar so that I would not forget something that might have some importance later.

John was having trouble sleeping all night. Some nights he was awake up to 20 times a night. This problem had been going on for about a year. Other times he was up, sitting on the side of the bed but he would not be awake. There were a few occasions when he had fallen out of bed, or he slipped as he would try to make his way to the washroom.

I was not sleeping most of the time, because I felt someone had to watch over him to make sure he was alright.

I was feeling exhausted most of the time, but I had learned to cope with it for the most part, but now the stress of wondering what was going on with him was making things harder for me.

I called the Doctor's office in Campbellford, and the nurse made us an emergency appointment when she heard what was happening. I could hear her on the computer typing and then she said, "Would 4 pm. today be good for you?"

We sat in the Doctor's office waiting for him to finish with a patient and then see John. A few minutes later the door opened, and Dr Read walked in with a smile on his face.

"Hello John, how are you feeling today?"

Slowly John glanced up at the Doctor, and then it seemed with great effort he said, "I've had better days."

"Well explain to me what is happening."

Once again John was slow in his response and finally said, "I can't see to read anything anymore. I can't see the TV, and I don't understand what they are talking about anyway." He hesitated as if he was thinking about something else to say but then sat back and looked at the Doctor.

I spoke up at this point and said, "John has had distortions where his perception of people's faces is cartoon-like because the features are all distorted."

"Tell me, John, how often is this happening?"

Again, John hesitated and then said slowly, "I guess the distortions are a couple of times a day." Then he looked at me as if to verify his response.

I smiled at him and shook my head yes.

"Do you have any headaches?" Dr Read inquired.

"Not that I remember."

"Is there anything else that you feel or see?"

John looked at the Doctor and said, "I feel weak a lot of the time."

"How is the Parkinson Medication working for you? Has it helped with any of the pain that you were experiencing? We had increased the dose for you trying to help with some of the pain. Do you think it has done anything for the tremor?"

"I think it is helping with the pain and yes maybe with the tremor as well," John responded slowly.

Dr Read went onto his computer and typed in the symptoms of what John was feeling. While he was doing that, I explained the information on the rare brain disease called Prosopometamorphosia. "It is supposed to be a disease that the patient sees people's faces distorted and cartoon-like. John has been saying that he sees an eye missing or a nose in the wrong place or mouth where an eye should be."

"I've never heard of this before, and I would like to read some more about it," said Dr Read. "Well, since we are going to be closed for the Christmas season, I will spend some time researching this, and we will meet back here in the New Year.

Let us see how things are going, and decided what we should do. I will increase your Parkinson medication.

CHAPTER 2

A few days later I was sitting in the kitchen while the children Vince and Alyssa were playing outside. I got up and put my coat on and went out to see what they were up too.

"Hey guys," I called out seeing them standing in the snow at the side of the house. "What are you two doing?"

They both turned around, and Vince called out, "We found some bubbles under the bench on the deck, and we are sending bubbles up to heaven with a prayer in it."

I was so surprised to hear this. "What kind of prayers are you sending in a bubble to Heaven?"

"We are praying that our house will be ready in time for Christmas to make Mommy and Daddy extremely happy." They both seemed to answer at the same time.

"That is such a wonderful idea," I called back to them. "How about some hot chocolate when you're finished."

"We'll be in soon." They both called out again.

I walked back into the house very touched that they would even think about doing something like that.

Adrian and Natalia had both gone to work. They were finding it very hard to live at my house and make the hour's drive to get to work and then another hour to get back again. At first, they stayed in a motel with the kids for a couple of days, but it was too crowded and uncomfortable. At least this way they all had a home environment and more space.

About three days later, they received word that they could move in on the weekend. They were all excited and happy to finally be in their own home for Christmas they were all smiling and trying to pack things back up again to take to their new house.

"Your prayers in the bubbles you sent up to Heaven worked," I said smiling at the twins.

The Christmas season was busy with Adrian and Natalia and the kids moving out of our house and into their new home. I was happy for them to be able to be in their own home for the Holiday season, but at the same time, I hated to see them go.

I feel so alone now; I thought to myself as I walked into the house after helping them move some of their things in my SUV. I had no one around anymore that I could get to help me with John if I suddenly needed help.

The house was suddenly quiet. Too quiet I thought to myself, I need sound and I went to the TV and turned it on.

We were sitting in the living room the second night after they had moved out and John was watching TV. "I don't understand what they are talking about on the TV. It's all gibberish. What's wrong with these TV shows and the news is no better. Even the commercials don't make any sense anymore."

"Well, why don't we turn it off and put some music on," I suggested as I got up and grabbed the TV converter and changed the channel to a Christmas music channel.

John got up from his chair and sauntered into the kitchen. He dropped his cane on the floor, and it fell with a bang.

I jumped up off the sofa with my heart in my throat as I thought he had fallen and was relieved to see he was alright but standing and staring at this cane lying on the floor. I walked over and picked it up and handed it to him.

"I wonder how that got there." He said as he took hold of it.

"Can I get you anything?" I asked.

"I would like new glasses because I can't even read a book with these. Where are my old glasses? I want them? They have to be better than these."

I looked around the house and found a couple of old pairs that he had, and he tried them all on and could not make up his mind if one pair was any better than another pair.

He went back to his chair in the living room and wanted to try and watch TV again.

"Could you put the movie back on for me? I want to see if I can see it now with these glasses," John said.

I picked up the converter and changed the channel. I usually did anyway as we had discovered that John had a hard time to push buttons because of the tremor and usually knocked the satellite out when he tried to change the channel. I sat down on the sofa and just watched him. I could see the frustration on his face as he tried to understand what was on the TV.

"Did you see that?"

"See what?" I asked.

"Oprah Winfrey was just on the screen, and she has her nose in her eye. Did you see that?"

"No, I can't see what you see," I replied sadly. My heart was in my throat as I observed John. I felt like my breathing had changed and I just wanted to take the distorted images away from him and make everything alright.

"Look," he said pointing to the TV. "That man has no eyes at all. He has black holes where his eyes should be. Do you see that?"

"Let's just put the music back on again," I said as I picked up the converter.

"No, I want to watch TV if you don't mind."

"Not at all, I am going to go in my office and get some paperwork done," I said calmly.

I got up from the sofa and went into my office. I sat in my chair and within a few minutes, tears were streaming down my face. I felt so scared, as I did not know what to expect next.

I picked up the phone and called Adrian. The phone rang twice, and then I heard his voice on the phone.

"Adrian, I just needed to hear a friendly voice. John is confused and thinks I should be seeing the same things that he is seeing. Meaning the distortions etc., he is seeing things a lot tonight."

"Yes, it's got to be hard," Adrian stated. "I know that he is having a hard time, but I question what is going on with him. It is hard to know what is wrong when it involves the brain, as it can be so many things. Whatever this is, it is getting worse."

"We are going back to the Doctor in a few more days, and I hope we get to the bottom of this soon. It scares me when I see that he is getting worse."

"Be strong, and if you need to call me in the middle of the night, please do. You can call anytime. We will do whatever we can."

We said our goodbyes a few minutes later, and I hung up. I went into the living room and found John dozing in his chair. I tapped him lightly on his shoulder, and he opened his eyes and smiled.

"Your mouth is in your eye," he said sleepily.

"Oh you are a charmer," I smiled back. "You always know the right thing to say to a woman."

He looked at me a little confused, and I just smiled again at him and then said, "How about we make it an early night and go to bed and get some rest? I'll take the dogs out, and then we can get ready for bed."

"Sounds good," he said as he started to get up out of his chair.

"Stay there," I said until I get the dogs walked and then I'll come and get you."

"Alright," he said as he sat back down.

I rushed getting my coat on and taking the dogs out for a quick pee just on the front lawn. Then I went back inside. I turned the TV off and turned all the lights off except the hallway and then I tapped John on the shoulder as he had fallen asleep in his chair again. He opened his eyes.

"I'm ready if you are," I said trying to sound light-hearted.

"Sure," he said as he attempted to get up.

I stepped forward and took hold of his arm and then guided him up out of the chair. He stood still for a couple of minutes as if trying to gain his composure. He swayed a few times, and I stood still beside him holding onto his arm and bracing my feet so that I could grab him if he started to fall.

Eventually, he seemed to get strong enough and took a few unsteady steps towards the hallway and the stair lift.

During the night he was very restless, and he was up and down 14 times. He would sit up on the side of the bed in his sleep. He would stay like that for about fifteen minutes and then he would lie back down again. Other times he would get up and go down the hall to the washroom, and a few minutes later he would be back. He would sit on the side of the bed and fall asleep, and I would wake him up and try to get him to lie down and relax. It seemed that this was becoming the norm. He would do this almost every night. I was averaging about 2 to 3 hours of broken sleep a night. Exhaustion was just a mild way of putting how I felt. There were times now that I would feel sick to my stomach from being so tired.

The next day he seemed a bit better until about three o'clock in the afternoon, and then he began to talk about the distorted faces he saw on the TV. Around six O'clock in the evening I was in the kitchen cleaning up from dinner. John walked in and stood beside the counter and gave me a strange look.

I smiled at him and asked, "How are you feeling?"

"I feel fine," he responded, "But the dog looks like a swamp person."

My heart sank. I felt an instant panic that seemed to knock the breath out of me. Trying to sound relaxed and not show how I was feeling, I took a big breath and said softly, "Which dog looks like a swamp person?"

"That one there," he said as he pointed to the small brown dog that we had rescued about a year ago.

Still trying to sound casual, I said, "Oh you mean Ace?"

"Yes, that one, that dog looks like a person living in a swamp."

"Oh, well," I stammered as I tried to think of some logical statement to make, but my mind had completely turned to mush. "Ace could use a bath I suppose."

"That's not going to help," John said slowly.

"Well, what do you think will help?" I asked

"Maybe a coffee," John said as he started to walk out of the kitchen.

"I'm not sure that the dog likes coffee," I said smiling trying to lighten the moment.

John just gave me a look and walked into the living room.

With raised eyebrows I watched him walk away, and I whispered to myself, "Maybe a coffee." I gave a big sigh as I poured the water into the coffee maker.

I handed him a coffee, with a piece of cake that I had made to take to Adrian and Natalia's house for Christmas the next day.

I still had some gifts to wrap, and I usually enlisted John to do the wrapping for me.

He was always so meticulous about doing a good job. He would spend hours matching up the design on the paper and trying to use only one or two small pieces of tape. So, I thought this might be good for him. Get him doing something that he likes doing.

I went and got the wrapping paper and scissors and tape and turned on some Christmas music and then retrieved the gifts that still needed wrapping.

"Hey John," I said as I walked by with my arms full of gifts. "How about coming into the kitchen and helping me wrap some gifts? You know you are so good at wrapping presents. Christmas isn't Christmas if I don't watch you wrap gifts."

He gave me a confused look and then realized what I had just said,
"Alright, I can do that for you."

He struggled to get up out of his chair but finally managed and then slowly followed me into the kitchen.

I laid everything down on the table and then guided him to a chair. I handed him the paper, scissors and tape and a gift. Then I grabbed a gift and another pair of scissors and some wrapping paper. "We have to share the tape," I said smiling.

He looked up and smiled at me and then he proceeded to try and wrap a gift. He put a small square box on the paper and turned it one way and then another. He picked up the box and looked at it closer and then placed the box back onto the paper. He again turned it one way and then another. He put it on its side and then rolled it over and over and over.

He attempted to put the wrapping paper over it, and then he turned the box around and placed the paper over it again. The wrapping paper was getting wrinkled, and the more he fought with it, the more twisted it became, and the more I could see his frustration grow.

I wrapped two boxes and then I got up and got a drink of water. "Would you like something to drink?"

"Not right now," he said almost absentmindedly as he concentrated on doing the job. He twisted the box inside the paper that he was holding over it. He grabbed the tape dispenser and started fighting with it. He put the box back down on the table, and all of his concentration went onto the tape. He tried to break a piece off but to no avail. Then he picked up the scissors and decided to cut a piece of tape off, but that didn't work. Next, he tried to bite a portion of the tape off, but it got stuck in his beard. With the dispenser hanging off his face he acted like he had forgotten it was there, and John put his concentration back onto the box he was wrapping. He put his hand on the gift and twisted the paper around the present. Now he had a mass of twisted paper wrapped around the present and no tape.

"Would you like some help?" I asked as I looked at John sitting there with a jumbled mass of Christmas paper with a tiny box that had now managed to disappear inside this massive mound of red, white, and green wrapping.

He looked at me with the tape dispenser hanging from his beard and the stress of the last few days caught up with me.

It was either laugh or cry, and I burst into laughter and could not stop. Tears rolled down my face as I tried to regain my composure.

It took a few minutes, and finally, I managed to say, "Here let me break some tape off for you," and I reached over and gently removed the tape dispenser from his beard. "I will put a few pieces on the table beside you, and you can take them as you need them."

He put a piece of tape over the box without any paper attached to it. Then he grabbed another piece of tape and put it on the paper but nowhere near the gift. He then pushed the wrapping into one end of the gift box and put tape on it, taping the paper to the inside of the box.

I stood back and leaned up against the counter and watched. It broke my heart to see this man who was once an air force machinist, now not knowing how to gift wrap a square box.

"If you've had enough I can finish this," I said trying to give him a way out if he wanted.

"No I want to do this," he said with determination in his voice.

About two hours later John sat back and said, "I have completed the wrapping." The square gift was wrapped with a complete roll of paper attached to it. "What do you think?"

"Well," I said choosing my words carefully, "I think you need a break. You put a lot of effort into that one. You do throw yourself completely into your work," I smiled. "It's getting late, and we can get ready for bed. I'll finish these later."

Christmas day came, and I loaded up the car, and we made our way to Church.

We met Adrian, Natalia and the kids there. We sat in the pews and listened to the beautiful Christmas message. I felt at peace when I was in the Church. I prayed that John would have a Christmas miracle and start to feel alright again.

After the service, we went back to Adrian's house for a delicious meal and watched the kids open their gifts. I was amazed that the children had such control. Most kids would wake up on Christmas morning and rush to unwrap everything at once. Natalia and Adrian had taught the kids to respect the true meaning of Christmas and wait until after Church to open their gifts.

Snow fell all day continuously and around 4 pm. I thought we had better hit the road before we got snowed in completely.

As we drove through one of the smaller towns, on our way home, I saw that there was a variety store up ahead that was open. "How about I stop and get you a chocolate bar or something to nibble on since we have a long drive ahead of us. I want to take my time because of the road conditions so that it will make our trip even longer."

"That sounds like a good idea," John responded.

I pulled into the parking lot just as another car drove in as well. They stopped first, and a couple of people jumped out and ran into the store.

I got out and went around and assisted John who was struggling to get his feet out on the ground.

"Watch your step it's slippery out here," I said as I neared the car door.

We made it to the door of the store and then John seemed to lose his footing and slipped through the door. He staggered a bit and then managed to regain his footing.

"Are you alright?" I asked.

John just shook his head, yes and we carried onto the candy counter.

I could see out of the corner of my eye that the people who had entered the store just before us were now standing back and watching us. They seemed to be whispering. I felt anger at what I knew they were thinking. I thought about saying something and then changed my mind.

John grabbed a chocolate bar and a drink, and we made our way to the counter where we paid and left the store.

I assisted John back to the car and then into his seat. I then went around and got in the driver's side. Just as I started the car, I heard a big sigh out of John.

I looked over at him, and he was visibly upset.

"Are you alright?"

"No. Sometimes it bothers me when people stare at me because they think I'm drunk. Other times it doesn't bother me at all about what they are thinking. Today it is bothering me. I know they all thought that I'm drunk."

"If they are that ignorant to think that, then they are not worth getting upset about," I said smiling.

"Deep down I know you are right, but it doesn't make it any easier," John replied.

"Think about it for a moment; if they don't know that an illness can cause someone to stumble, then they still have a lot to learn in life and chances are they will not be able to handle it if something should happen to them. People like that will stumble many times in life, and in reality, they have just made a stumble by not recognizing someone who is not drunk."

"That's true," he said sadly.

"Look at the nice snowy scenery out your window and forget about them. How about you being my navigator and tell me when I'm driving in a farmer's field instead of on the road, since I can't tell where the road is because of all of this white stuff," I smiled and then started the car and made my way back onto the road again.

The snow falling was getting thicker, and I had to concentrate on staying on the road. In places, it was hard to know where the white line was on the street because of the whiteout conditions. I was not sure where I was at some points. What was an hour's drive turned into two and a half hours. I turned Christmas music on and just took my time. We only passed about four cars the entire way home.

John was quiet for most of the drive. If I said something, sometimes he would respond, and other times he just stayed quiet.

When we got home, I made a quick sandwich and gave him his medications. I was grateful that he never lost his appetite no matter how he felt, he was always hungry.

I assumed that it had something to do with the fact that he was burning a lot of energy with the tremor and therefore he was hungry most times.

Later we were sitting in the living room, and he said, "I am having different visions now."

"What type of different visions?"

"When I look at a flat surface like a wall or a counter I see what looks like fish scales. Sometimes they are moving, but most of the time they are just there."

"Are you seeing this on people's faces as well?"

"No, only on flat surfaces," he responded.

"How long has this been happening?"

"A couple of days now," he answered.

"Why wouldn't you tell me before this?"

"I don't know, but I'm telling you now."

"Well I am keeping track of what you are experiencing, and I want you to tell me things when they are happening so that I can write them down. Please remember that it is important to me to try and keep track of what is happening." I said trying not to sound alarmed.

I just wanted it all to stop. I could not understand how something like this could be happening. How did John get a rare brain disease? I felt despair because I was not sure what else was going to happen.

"I'm tired, and I think I will go to bed," he said.

"Sounds like a great idea," I responded.

About an hour later I lay in bed beside him and listened to his deep breathing. I was always fascinated with the fact that when he would fall asleep, the tremor would instantly stop. And as soon as he would begin to wake up the shaking would start up again.

I had read somewhere that many people with a tremor or Parkinson's disease would drink because it would stop the shaking for a short time. I had discussed it with John, and he said that it was true. He had done it years ago and found that it was helpful only for a few hours, but there was always payback later because the tremor would be worse the next day. He has had an Essential tremor since he was about 16 years of age. It just got progressively worse over the years. When he was told he had Parkinson's one of the Doctor's said, "Just because you now have Parkinson's does not mean that the Essential Tremor is suddenly gone, it means you have both."

Throughout the night John awoke about every 20 minutes. He was uncomfortable, and he was restless. Even in his sleep, John was still getting up. He would sit on the side of the bed and continue to sleep and then he would lie back down for about 20 minutes and then he would get up and sit there again. Now and then he would get up and go down the hallway to the washroom and then come back again. Finally, around 5 am., he settled down and went to sleep and stayed that way without moving until about 8 am.

I fell into an exhausted sleep.

We awoke to a world covered in white crystals. The tree branches were laden with ice. They were so heavy that they were bending with the weight. All of the houses around were shimmering with the sun glistening off the ice that covered them, and the street had a sparkling crystal finish to it that looked like someone could skate on, if they wished.

"It looks so pretty out there," I said as I got ready to take the dogs out. "Instead of putting boots on to take the dogs for a walk I should put skates on instead," I smiled as I grabbed my coat and then put the leashes on the two little dogs.

I walked outside to find that it was slippery. I took a couple of steps and then I held onto the railing of the deck and slowly made my way to the end and then carefully I went down each step until finally, I was standing on the ground. The dogs had a hard time to walk, and their little feet were slipping out from underneath them. The white miniature poodle stood up and put her feet two front feet onto my leg and begged to be picked up. I bent down and retrieved her, and she snuggled down into my red plaid coat, soaking up as much warmth as she could. She never did really like winter.

Ace, the little brown dog, was a bit more adventurous. He struggled with his footing on the ice, but he was determined that he was going to go for his walk. Both dogs are rescues, and they had been through a lot in their lives. It was nice to see them come out of their shells after they had been living with us for a while. Leo the larger dog was slipping and sliding around in his pen and I looked over just in time to see his four feet slide out from underneath him and he went sliding across the ground on his stomach with four legs stretched out to his sides, just like Bambi did in the movie. I laughed as I stood there and watched him.

He struggled to get up, and three times in a row he would fall back down with his legs sprawled out from under him each time. Finally, he got the hang of how to stand and carefully got up and made his way slowly to the gate to wait for me to retrieve him.

A few minutes later we were all back in the house, and they were eating their breakfast, and I gave John his medications and then poured him a coffee. He sat eating his breakfast, and I sat down sipping on a coffee as well.

"So is it cold outside?" John asked.

"No, it's lovely out there. When I was outside, I felt like I was standing in the middle of a big ice painting. You can see the strokes of the brush on the trees making designs and patterns on the windows and doors," I said, "I heard the weather a little while ago, and they are calling for more snow today and tonight."

I looked over at John and was surprised to see that he had his fried egg sandwich in his hand halfway to his mouth. His mouth was partially open, and he was sound asleep.

I just sat there watching him, wondering how he could fall asleep in the middle of eating.

He stayed like that for about 4 minutes and then he suddenly woke up. He took a bite of his sandwich and then in the middle of chewing he seemed to fall back asleep again.

"John," I called out to him. "Do you want to go back to bed?"

"No, I just got up," he responded.

"Alright, I just thought I'd ask," I smiled.

That day he had about 14 visions that he talked about seeing. They were becoming more frequent, and there were times that he would think that I should see them as well. He also spoke about how the textured surfaces on the counters in the kitchen or washrooms where all are looking like fish scales.

"I also see things tipped on their sides," John said. "Remember a few years ago when I saw things tipped in your office? I would tell you that a cup on your desk looked like it was on an angle? Well, that is what I see now also."

He sat down that evening in the living room and tried watching a few different TV shows. "I don't understand what anyone is talking about in the commercials or the movie. It just sounds like gibberish. I want to read a book, but I can't see the words on the pages. I want to build something or do something, but I can't see to do anything. Not being able to hear properly or see things is frustrating. Why can't I get a pair of glasses to suit my eyes?"

I did not know how to respond to any of what he was saying. So I tried to choose my words carefully, but they sounded empty to me, so I'm sure they did to him as well. "We will just have to keep trying to find a way to get you a pair of glasses that will suit you."

John looked at me, and I could see the exasperation and frustration on his face.

"How about we just turn some music on again?"

I got up from my seat and got the TV converter and put on a 50's music channel and began to sing to the song that was playing. It was an old time classic of Elvis Presley,

John smiled and seemed to relax a bit.

"How about some of that chocolate cake that I made this afternoon?" I asked.

He moved towards the table, and I noticed that he was having a hard time to sit down. The kitchen table was glass, and I realized that he was having a hard to see the glass on the table top.

"Do you have a hard time seeing this table?" I inquired.

"Yes, I can't tell where the edge of the table is. I have to reach out and touch it to know where it is. I walk into it sometimes, and when I go to sit down, I have to touch the table first to know exactly where it is."

I got up and took a table cloth out of a drawer in the kitchen and put it on the table. "Maybe this will help."

"It should," he smiled as he munched away on his piece of cake.

I watched him for the next few days and realized that the cloth on the table was not working. It was now just one more thing that he had to deal with, which only made matters worse. He would try to sit down, and the table cloth would fall to the floor. He would try to stand up from the table, and the fabric would start sliding and go with him. I was worried that he was going to trip on it.

"I have thought that I would like to build an island here in the kitchen," I said one morning as we sat at the table sipping on our coffee. "It would give me more working space, and it would also give me more storage. I think it would be good for you too because we can get bar stools that would be higher and then it will be easier for you to sit down or stand up. These chairs are too low for you with your long legs. You are always struggling to get off these chairs once you sit down. So what do you think?"

"If you want," John said. "It might be nice to have an island."

Later that morning we went shopping at Habitant for Humanity store, and I found an old sideboard that had drawers on each side of a stained glass door that I could make into an elegant and unique island. It had shelves in the middle for added storage. I can turn this into a beautiful island for the kitchen. We have to order a countertop to go on top.

I gave the table and chairs away. I felt that the sooner the glass table was out of the kitchen, the better, as there were a few times that he looked like he was going to fall through the table because of not being able to judge where the glass was.

The day came that the delivery of the sideboard and countertop arrived. I stood back and wondered how I was going to do this since I had never made anything in my life like this. Carpentry was not something that I had ever attempted before, but I knew how I wanted this to look, and I was going to make it happen somehow.

I needed to raise the height of the counter so that it would be the same size as the other counters in the kitchen.

I decided that I could put 2x4x8 on the top and paint it the same as the other counters in the kitchen. Then I would have to put the countertop onto this and fasten it down.

Two days and a lot of struggle later I stood back and admired what was now my first Island job. It looked professional, and I was pleased with how it suited the kitchen. The stools that I had purchased to go with the counter had swivel seats so that John would find it easy to get on or off them.

That night John sat in the kitchen and had a bowl of cereal. I prepared the dogs food as they always ate around ten at night and then I would take them for a quick walk. As I worked at getting their meal together, I asked John, "So are you finding it easier to sit on the taller chairs rather than regular table chairs?"

"I think that I…" he stopped talking.

I waited a moment and then turned around from the food preparation and looked at him and was surprised to see that he had the spoon in his hand and almost halfway to his mouth and his mouth was partially open. He looked like someone frozen in time as he was sound asleep. I stood there and just watched him amazed how someone could fall asleep like that.

CHAPTER 3

"I guess they are alright," he said as he looked into the mirror and turned his head from one angle to another, looking at his new eyeglasses. He read several lines from a piece of paper they handed him, and he acknowledged that he thought the glasses where alright.

We left the Optical store and went to have lunch at a local fish restaurant called Jeff Purveys. We always enjoyed going there any time we went into Peterborough. "I think they have the best fish in town," John said as he ate his meal. "The staff here is friendly and easy to talk too. I feel welcomed every time we walk through the door."

When we left the restaurant, we went to do some shopping. While we were in a store looking around, there was a man in an aisle trying to get a signal on his cell phone. The gentleman continued to yell into the phone, "Hello, hello," and then he would go to another spot in the store and try it again.

He repeated this four or five times without much success on getting a stronger signal.

John was leaning on his cane and watching the man in amusement. Finally, without any warning, John yelled out loudly in the store in a slow country drawl, "Can you hear me now?!"

I looked at John who stood with a small smirk on his face. The other people in the store stopped what they were doing and looked at John. Many of them started laughing. The man with the phone smiled and walked out of the store. The stress and tension came to the surface for me, and I began to laugh. The more I tried to stop laughing the worse it got. Tears ran down my face, and I had to leave the store and look for a washroom, with John following behind me, still with the same little smirk on his face.

A couple of days later John started complaining that the glasses were not working right.

"They must have gotten the prescription wrong," he said, "I keep seeing things that look out of place. Things seem to be distorted, and I still see a glass on a counter sitting on an angel and when I walk through a door the step down is out of focus."

"Well let's go back and see what they can do."

The next day we went back and explained what John was seeing. "We don't know what is wrong. The prescription is fine. It matches what your eyes need. It's fine here and then a few days after you leave you are having problems again. It's not the glasses. We don't know what it is but to keep changing the glasses is not working."

John was frustrated and so was I as we left the office. "What am I supposed to do?"

"We'll just make another appointment with someone else, and we will keep looking until we get some answers," I promised.

So we made an appointment with another Optometrist, and they said the same thing. "We don't believe that your eyes are the problem. There must be something else happening," the Doctor said.

"Is there nobody that knows how to do their job anymore?" John asked in frustration.

"I am amazed," I said. "I don't know what to think."

At the same time, John's tremor was getting worse. The distortions he was seeing where increasing daily. He had gone from seeing just a few a day to now seeing about ten or twelve a day. He was acting more and more confused, and it was hard for him to carry on a conversation. We would be talking about something and then suddenly he would start to say something in response and forget what he was talking about and just become quiet.

I could see the frustration growing, but at the same time, he still would try to keep his sense of humour.

"I think that some of these distortions of people's faces can be an improvement when you are looking at a Politician on the TV giving a speech. I see their ear where their mouth should be," he said smiling as he looked at something on the TV set.

"I have to say that I do admire you as you are accepting this much better than I ever would. You are an inspiration to me as I would be crying and acting like an insane person by now if I was having these distortions like you are."

John just smiled and said, "The distortions are not bad really. The visions don't bother me as much as not being able to read. I find it more frustrating that I can't see a book. If we can get my eyes fixed, then I will feel a lot better about everything."

"Well, we will just have to keep trying until we do."

"I will call and sit up another appointment with your family Doctor Read and see if he can send us to my eye specialists in Peterborough, as she is amazing. Remember she operated on my eyes when I had gotten glaucoma and saved my eyesight a few years ago and if anyone can help, I'm sure she can."

That afternoon we sat in the office of Doctor Read.

"I want you to talk as I get confused a lot," said John as we waited for Doctor Read to come into the examining room.

A few minutes later the Doctor arrived and sat down. He smiled at John and asked, "So how is it going?"

"John still has the distortions, and he also is still having a hard time to try and see or read things." I tried to explain. "Everything still looks out of proportion for him, and this makes it difficult, not just for reading but also for walking through doorways etc... we would like to see if we could get an appointment with my eye specialists in Peterborough."

"I don't know if she is going to be able to help with this. It might be more a brain issue rather than an eye issue," Dr Read responded.

"We know that, but we would like to explore all avenues if we can. So if you could recommend John to her, maybe we can get him seen and go from there with her findings."

"I have no problems with John going to see her, so yes I will fill out the paperwork, and hopefully they will contact you soon," said Dr Read smiling at John. "How is the pain?"

"I still have some, but I think it might be a bit better," replied John.

"We have been increasing your Parkinson's medication, so I think we will continue to increase the dosage and put you on six times a day now and see how you feel."

That night as I was preparing dinner, I said to John, "I don't understand what has happened to all of my sharp knives. There is only two left in the drawer. They seem to be missing. Have you seen them?"

"No, I don't know where they are. Most people complain of missing socks, but you have missing knives."

"Yes, it seems strange that they could just suddenly go missing," I said perplexed.

The next morning I was going to Johns shed to look for a screwdriver that he took and used over there? When I opened the door, I saw that my missing knives where all on the floor of the shed sitting beside a knife sharpener.

When I went back into the house, I said, "John I found my missing knives in your shed sitting beside a knife sharpener."

"That's right. I forgot about that. I was going to sharpen the knives, but I never got around to it." He smiled and said, "I'll do it now."

"Alright if you want to but if you can't just bring them back in so that I will have some knives in the kitchen."

About an hour later he walked in with all of my knives and handed them to me and said you could try them and see if they are sharp.

I tried them all, and some were, and some were not, but I smiled and said, "They are great. Thanks, I appreciate that very much."

That evening my sister called around 6 pm. and said that she was watching TV and a commercial came on, and she wondered if I had ever seen it. "It was an ad for dementia. A man standing, and he thought he saw a ghost, and he started talking to this ghost. Then the commercial went onto say that this type of thing happens with dementia.

"No, I have never seen it. I hope that it comes on again so that I can. What did it say?"

"I'm not sure. I wasn't paying that much attention to it until it was almost over and then I realized what the commercial was talking about someone seeing things that are not there. Then they talked about dementia. So I wondered if it could be what John is experiencing," she replied.

That night I sat down at the computer and typed in dementia and read as much as I could about it. I didn't think that it was what John was experiencing as it talked about seeing people that are not there and losing reality in certain situations. John did not see dead people. He does grasp the reality of what is happening around him. He is always aware of his surroundings.

I began calling the things he saw, distortions and not visions. There is a difference I said to John. A vision is something that you see that is not there. A distortion is something that is there but out of place, such as an eye where a mouth should be.

For the next few weeks, we waited patiently for an appointment with the eye specialist. During that waiting period, John's struggle with the distortions continued to get even worse. He was getting up about fifteen times a night now, and he was slowly drifting away from me mentally.

He was with me and then suddenly not and then with me again and then suddenly not. It is like a rollercoaster that we were on, and the highs and lows were now a part of our everyday.

We would be having conversations, and then he would stop talking as if he was thinking the rest of the sentence instead of saying it. I would watch him waiting to see if he would come back and finish, but most times he did not.

Fear and frustration on my part grew daily. I did not know what to expect most of the time. He would decide to do things and maybe get some tools and bring them into the kitchen or living room and then leave them laying there on a counter or beside his chair and never touch them again.

I would eventually pick them up a few days later and put them back in their place. He would not remember why he had gotten them out.

I found him on several occasions just standing and looking out a window. I could tell that he did not see anything.

I was cleaning the kitchen after breakfast one morning, and he walked into the kitchen and took a chair and sat down facing the window. He sat there for a long time. I didn't say anything but just watched him as I cleaned. It was as if he had not noticed me in the kitchen. Finally, I asked him, "So what are you watching?"

He turned his head and looked at me and then asked, "Watching?"

"Yes, what are you watching out the window?"

"I didn't know I was watching anything out the window," he said as he got up and walked into the living room.

"Well, I need you to get ready as we have your Chiropractic treatment today. It's an hour drive, so we need to leave soon" I called out to John as he walked away.

"Today we have to go?"

"Yes so let's get ready," I replied.

I still took him for his chiropractor treatments and for the most part I felt that they worked a bit for him. It was not a cure by any means, but I believe that they were helping to keep him mobile and moving.

He would stand a little straighter and taller for a few days after the treatments. He would walk better even though he still complained of the pain. Dr Cocek was fantastic with John understanding that he was in tremendous pain and they would fit him into a schedule so that he would not have to sit and wait for his treatments. The office staff schedule John to be the first patient seen after lunch, and we appreciated it. The office staff were terrific with him as they always had a smile and made sure that the office atmosphere was light and enjoyable.

The rest of the day he complained of having the distortions about fifteen times. We were in the car driving home from the Chiropractor, and John started mentioning that the sides of the road where distorted.

"That's alright," I said trying to sound light-hearted. "It must make the snow more interesting."

"I guess you could look at it that way," he said looking out the window.

John was sent for an MRI and brain scans at the Cobourg Hospital the next day, and the results were back within a couple of days.

We received a phone call from the Doctors office asking up to come in and get the results.

"Where the plaque is growing on the brain and with the symptoms that John has, it leads us to believe that he has Lewy Body," said Dr Read. "It is hard to diagnose it until after a person dies and an autopsy has been performed."

"I think I'll pass on that test," John said as he heard the news.

"It's nice to see that you continue to smile," said Dr Read as we left his office.

When we got home, there was a message on the answering machine. It was just a coincidence, but a friend of ours called and left me a message on the phone telling me that she had looked up what she thought might be happening to John and she also came up with the name of the disease called Lewy Body and wanted me to look into it and see what I thought.

I called her back that night and said, "Wow you are good. The Doctor just gave us the news that the ex-rays and tests show that John has Lewy Body as far as they can tell. With all of the symptoms and tests results the Doctor feels that it is a strong possibility that this is the disease he is suffering from."

A few days later we sat in the eye specialists office in Peterborough, and we watched people come and go. The place was full of patients, and everyone seemed happy to be there. They all knew they were seeing one of the best Ophthalmologists in Peterborough and if they had to sit and wait for a few hours that were fine with them.

The office had some hockey memorabilia hanging on the walls and a few paintings. A TV was sitting up against a far wall with the news and weather rolling on the screen. For the most part, the office was light and airy with windows all across one wall, which overlooked the Peterborough Hospital.

Finally, John got escorted into the examining room. With not much effort they ordered some tests to be done right then.

John went to get the tests done which did not take more than ten minutes and then he was back waiting to see the eye specialists. A little while later the Doctor sat at her desk in front of John and looked at the results from the tests just performed. Then she put drops in his eyes and examined him. Within a couple of minutes, she sat back in her chair and said, "Alright John I see by the tests that we have done that you do have a crater behind your left eye. That crater is filling up with fluid, and that is what is giving you the distortions."

I could not believe what I was hearing. I felt this flood of relief flow over me, and I could feel tears well up in my eyes as she continued.

"I want you to see a Doctor in Oshawa as she is terrific and she does this type of surgery. She may be able to help you. You have a cataract on your eye as well, but I don't want to touch it until you have seen this Doctor and then let's see what she has to say."

John looked stunned as if he did not understand what she had just said.

I stood up and helped get him up out of the chair and handed him his cane. "Thank you so very much."

"Not a problem. Just give this to my nurse", as she handed me a piece of paper ", and she will sit up the appointment for you, and I will see you back here in about six weeks," then she stood up and directed us to the door.

Outside we stood in the parking lot and just digested the good news. "Wow! That means that you might get your sight back. You will be able to read and do all the things that you miss doing."

"I hope so. This eye problem has been frustrating; not being able to see things. So, what was it that the eye Doctor said that I have?"

"She called it a crater behind your left eye and as it fills up with fluid, and then you see things distorted."

I opened the car door and assisted him in. I handed him the seat belt and smiled as I closed the door and went around the car to the other side. I crawled in and sat there for a minute and laughed. "I am so happy for you. Now we have to wait to see this next Doctor."

As soon as we got back to the house, I called John's family Doctor and left him a message of the findings of the Ophthalmologist. We had another appointment with Doctor Read in a couple of days, but I thought he deserved the news then as he had been spending a lot of his free time doing research and trying to find answers for John as to what was happening and why.

Later that evening I was walking into the living room, and just as I entered through the doorway, I saw John make a motion with his hand that he was throwing something away. I was curious as I could not see anything. "What was that?" I asked.

"I was throwing away my cigarette before it burned my fingers." Then he smiled and giggled. "I don't know why but sometimes lately, I think I am holding a cigarette, and I toss it into an ashtray or onto the floor."

"Well since you quit smoking about eight years ago, I gave the ashtrays away.

So try not to burn the house down when you throw your cigarettes on the floor," I said smiling at him.

He laughed and said, "Alright I'll try not to." Then he proceeded to tell me that he has gone as far as putting his hand in his shirt pocket to retrieve a cigarette as that was where he used to carry them.

"How often do you think you're smoking?"

"Lately it has been a lot. I will even wake myself up tossing a cigarette away from me. We have been in the car, and I will think I'm smoking and attempt to throw it out the window."

"Well, I guess smoking was a huge part of your life at one point, and now for some strange reason your mind is recalling some of those moments."

CHAPTER FOUR

"Let's face it," I stated into the phone to my sister who was recovering from her husband's passing after being married 48 years. "It's tragic when anyone develops a terrible fatal disease."

"Yes, I agree," Laura stated sadly. "It's hard on the person who has the disease, and it's hard on the family members looking after someone who is ill."

"Robin Williams and Casey Kasem are a few people known to have or had Lewy Body Disease. Putting celebrity faces to the disease seems to help make people stop and listen to what it is all about," I stated.

"That's not surprising."

"I decided to look up to see what Lewy Body is all about, and much to my surprise, not a lot is known about it," I continued.

"Everything that I read seems to agree that many people have it but don't know that they do as it is often misdiagnosed. The disease was discovered in the early 1900s by a man called Friederich H.Lewy who was researching Parkinson's disease, and this was when he discovered that the abnormal protein deposits that disrupt the brain function. It is an umbrella term for the two related diagnoses, dementia with Lewy Bodies disease and Parkinson's."

Laura asked, "So, why is it so hard to diagnose?"

"Well if I understand correctly, it is not known for sure until an autopsy has been performed, but there are differences between Alzheimer's and Lewy body often referred to as LBD.

Alzheimer's patients have lapses of short term memory, which is some of the first symptoms for this disease.

LBD patients, on the other hand, encounter severe disruptions in attention and judgment. Sometimes with hallucinations, delusions, and severe disturbances in sleep, but these symptoms are not in Alzheimer's patients."

"Wow, it can be confusing," Laura commented. "So how can they diagnose John with Lewy Body?"

"Well after many attempts to diagnose it as other things and usually as in John's case, after seeing Doctors and having tests done it comes down to the symptoms that he is experiencing. John has most of the known symptoms associated with Lewy Body and also the results of the tests showing where he has the plaque buildup on the brain has helped to determine what he has.

Even with all the evidence pointing in the direction of Lewy Body, we will never really know for sure until after he has passed and an autopsy is completed."

"It is such a difficult disease; I guess that is why most people do not know about it."

"Yes, I agree with that," I said. "Also patients with LBD can be extra sensitive to certain medications."

"I've heard you are mentioning about how John has sleep disruptions and also about him not being able to take pain medications etc.," Laura said.

"Yes, your right, I have mentioned that," I agreed. "I also have read that for Alzheimer's patients the plaques that grow on the brain and tangles with proteins known as Beta-Amyloid and Tare. While Lewy Body is characterized by Lewy bodies Abnormal clumps of a protein called Alpha-Synuclein."

"Wow there is so much to learn about all of this," Laura stated.

"To make it even more confusing, the Doctor that did the autopsy on Robin Williams has stated that in many cases, people with Lewy Body are misdiagnosed. People with Parkinson's disease because the symptoms of having Lewy Body, can be about the same as having Parkinson's, but if a person who has Lewy Body is treated for Parkinson's medications can make the Lewy Body even worse," I said.

"Oh my God," Laura stated loudly into the phone. "Could this have happened in John's case?"

"I don't know for sure," I replied. "Patients with Lewy Body can hallucinate on their own, but when given Parkinson's medication then it can make the hallucinations worse. If that is what happened with John, it is so hard to say at this point. Remember with John, things get even a little more confusing as he also has the eye disease of having the crater behind his eye filling up with fluids and making things distorted."

"Oh yes, I had almost forgotten about that," said Laura, "With all of these other things happening, it is so hard to try and decipher what is happening."

"That's true," I carried on, "I'm beginning to think that the rough surfaces he sees and the glass sitting tipped, or the distorted step between a doorway is all due to the eye problem. The rest of the problems such as the visions of people having their faces distorted are a part of the hallucinations. He had stated one night that our little brown dog named Ace, looked like a swamp person. I believe these are all Lewy Body."

"That must be so hard on him to see this stuff and on you to see John go through it."

"I consider myself lucky that he is not afraid of the visions he has. He experiences no fearful emotions with anything. Instead, he finds it all rather amusing, and I am so grateful for that."

"Yes it could be a lot worse for you," Laura said. "He does have a good sense of humour, and he is always smiling for the most part, no matter how he feels.

Everyone that knows him knows that no matter how terrible he feels, or what kind of pain he has, he will always tell everyone when they ask him, "That he is great."

"Yes that's true, it has gotten to the point that most people that ask him how he is feeling, will now answer the question at the same time he does, saying "Great."

"He does have a good sense of humour, and that makes it easier for me. I still have a lot more to learn about Parkinson's and Lewy Body," I said, "I am disappointed that there is no Lewy Body chapter here in Canada. The most support that you can get for this disease is from the Alzheimer's Society which once again is different than Lewy Body. I have been in touch with Lewy Body organizations throughout Europe and also in the States, and they put me in touch with a gentleman in Toronto that runs a web site for Lewy Body.

"That's great, maybe he can give you some advice," Laura responded.

"I don't think so. The person running the web site said there is no funding to help run the site and he does not have a lot of time that he can put into the site."

"So what is on the site then?"

I tried of answering her question with, "Well it is there so that people can post on the site what their experience is with someone who has the disease. Caregivers can post their views, their fears, and what they have witnessed or what they go through as a caregiver. It was a bit helpful to read some of the posts from other people.

"I wonder why no one has started a Lewy Body Chapter here," Laura stated.

"I'm not sure, but someone has got to do it," I responded. "People need to be educated in this disease. We have a population that is getting older all the time. Some of the baby boomers are going to be suffering from this and not know they have it. Take a look at Robin Williams, he was diagnosed with Parkinson's, and he suffered from depression and had no idea why. He committed suicide before they knew what was wrong with him. Robin's wife believes that Lewy Body was the cause of him taking his own life."

"Is depression a part of this disease?" Laura asked.

"Yes it can be, and that is why it is so important that people know they are not alone when they have this. There needs to be more help for them. Think about the person that lives alone or has no family. How hard this must be for them."

"It's got to be terrible," Laura responded. "There should be more research into this disease."

"Well maybe once people start to recognize actors and actresses faces to the disease then maybe it will start to gain more interest and popularity. Right now the big dollars go to popular diseases such as cancer and heart and stroke. People will give big dollars to these diseases because they probably know someone who has the disease. Well, they probably know someone with this disease too, but they don't know it."

"Does the Doctor or anyone tell you where you can get some support?"

"No, not really, there is the support for Alzheimer's or Parkinson's diseases but not for Lewy body itself. Even though Lewy Body is a form of Dementia, it is still different. As you know with any illness, there is not much help out there for the custodial care and supervision required for someone with Parkinson's or dementia. No health care insurance will cover the cost of in-home care. The caregiver is responsible 24 hours a day, seven days a week. You can get a couple of hours off a week if you have the VON come in but that in itself can be very upsetting for someone with Lewy Body as I found out when I tried to have someone come in for three hours on Saturday's for John, so that I could go shopping or run errands. He was very uncomfortable with a stranger, and it would stress him out. They found him a high risk of falling and therefore they did not want him moving around a lot. So, I would put a movie on for him and make him lunch or a snack so that he had something while I was gone and try to make him as comfortable as possible, but instead, he was so uncomfortable that I cancelled them coming in after having it for only three weeks.

I heard Laura sigh and then say, "I agree with you that there is a need for a Lewy Body Chapter here in Canada. It's strange that not many people know much about this disease and most have never even heard of it."

"Yes, I was shocked by the fact that is it thought of to be the second most popular form of dementia but yet there is not much research being done on it."

"So what causes this or does anyone know?" Laura asked.

"Well, I know that there is the plaque buildup on the brain which happens to be the frontal lobe, which is the part of the brain that makes us human.

The frontal lobe is the part that is affected and makes this an incredibly devastating disease. It is attacking who you are as a person. It is taking you away piece by piece." My voice began to break with emotion. I took a big breath and tried to regain my composure. "I look at John, and there are times when we are talking and laughing, and then suddenly I see this blank look come into his eyes and I feel him begin to disappear. I want to take hold of him and beg him not to go."

"It's got to be hard for sure," Laura commented.

"Yes, it is. I feel that John's brain is becoming like a Torture Chamber. It takes him hostage and keeps him in the dark sometimes for a long length of time and other times it is only for a few minutes. There are times that I try to reach through and I can't break through the door when it closes," I said, as I wiped a tear away that ran down my face. I was so glad we were having this conversation over the phone so that she could not see my face or eyes.

"Yes, I have seen him on days when he is not totally with it. You can tell he tries so hard to understand what is going on, but there are moments you know he is not there," Laura stated.

"In the case of Robin Williams, he committed suicide before any real help could be given to him. He suffered depression, and it took a hold on him right away. Think about how many others have probably committed suicide over the years and did not know that they had Lewy Body. They probably just felt that their lives were out of control and they could not cope with the uncertainty." I said sadly.

"Yes it is sad that this disease even exists," Laura said.

"Well, then we have the case of Casey Kasem who was a big radio and TV personality. He has been diagnosed with this terrible disease as well. It is also a sad case."

"Oh no, not him too," Laura shouted into the phone. "That's terrible."

"Yes I agree, it is terrible," I replied. "It is proven that once this disease settles in, it is very hard on the patient to have any types of changes around them. That means that you have to try and keep things calm and peaceful as much as possible."

"Wow it must be devastating to the person who has this disease to try and get through their day," Laura exclaimed.

"Then there is the case of Tim Conway," I continued. "You remember him? He was famous for starring in the 1960's World War 11 sitcom, McHale's Navy and then the 1970's comedy The Carol Burnett Show."

Laura laughed and said, "Yes I remember him. Tim Conway had a wonderful sense of humour. I loved all of the shows I have ever seen him in,"

"Well, it is unfortunate what is happening to him. He has been diagnosed with some form of Dementia and is unable or unwilling to communicate, his lawyer, Michael Harris said. He shows no apparent signs that he comprehends the nature of anything that is happening."

"Yes, that is so sad," Laura responded.

"When I read about them, I wondered what other famous people have had some form of dementia.

There are big names on the list such as Charles Bronson, Charlton Heston, Perry Como, Rita Hayworth, Ronald Regan, Sugar Ray Robinson. Then there is my favorite artist Norman Rockwell, Bill Quakenbush a hockey player, Betty Schwartz who won a gold medal in track and field events, Paul Silva Henriquez a Roman Catholic Cardinal who fights for human rights and many, many more."

"Wow, I had no idea that it was prevalent."

"Yes it is widespread, and it knows no prejudice. It does not care about how wealthy or famous you are, and it doesn't care where you come from or the color of your skin, or your religion or your educational background. It can attack anyone at any time," I said sadly. "I have read that sometimes with the more advanced cases, the person will bear no resemblance to the person that you once knew."

"Oh my God," exclaimed Laura. "How on earth do the caregivers and families manage?"

"Well, a caregiver and family need to be bendable and be able to try and foresee what is going to happen. You can only do this if you are aware of their mood swings and be prepared that their moods can change drastically without a lot of warning. Also, because of these fluctuations, a person with this disease can become surprisingly agile and physical. Sometimes when you least expect it."

"My heart goes out to anyone experiencing this terrible disease," Laura stated. "Any form of dementia or Alzheimer's is devastating for the patient as well as the family."

"We have never had John experience any of those symptoms of mood swings, so far he is always smiling for the most part, or he becomes quiet and withdrawn for a while. I pray that we never do experience any of the mood swings. I have seen him go through what is termed freezing. Freezing is the temporary inability to move one's legs and feet. It has happened a few times now when he is getting in or out of a car. I have found that talking to him and just encouraging him to move his feet a certain way helps to get him going again."

"I had no idea what this disease could do to someone. Imagine most people have never even heard of it," Laura said.

"Yes, it attacks the autonomic nervous system that renders simple automatic reflexes difficult or ineffective. This means that swallowing can become a real danger. Also, it affects the blood pressure, heart rate fluctuations, incontinence and sleep disturbance. The unconscious mind has a problem telling the body what to do. Becoming aware of this meant that I had to watch what I was feeding John. And being right there or close by while he is eating.

"I had no idea how much responsibility you had to take on with this disease. It is a 24-hour watch. It is a full-time job," Laura stated.

"It is but I also am so very grateful that John is so easy going. It makes my life easier. He seems to accept everything for what it is and smiles. He tries so hard to make it easier on me," I replied.

"So have you ever recognized any real changes in his attitudes or likes or dislikes?" She asked.

"Actually, strange you ask that, "I have been thinking about the fact how strange it is that in the last few days that he has asked for a sandwich and each time he has wanted mayonnaise on it and yet all of the years I've known him, he never liked mayonnaise. He would purposely tell a restaurant or anyone making something for him to make sure that they did not put it on his food and here he is now asking for it."

"Wow, that's strange," Laura stated with surprise.

"Yes, I don't know why the change. I asked John the other day if he now likes mayonnaise and he just gave me a strange questioning look and never answered the question."

"Are there other things happening that you find unusual?"

"I'm to the point that I'm not sure what is unusual or what is now considered normal for his disease. In the last few days, he has been having double vision and flashing lights. He says that the lights are like the flash of a camera if you're taking a picture. So it comes and goes very quickly and never stays but it has been happening more frequently lately."

Laura said, "I admire him that he can go through all of this and not complain. Not get frustrated or get royally mad. Most people would get so upset by this happening to them."

"Yes, I agree," I stated. "If this were me I would probably be insane by now."

"He is amazing," Laura said.

"He talks a lot about things being tipped or sitting on an angle. He has been seeing things on an angle on and off for years.

He would mention it sometimes when I had my sign company, and he would be in the office. He would see things sitting on my desk as tipped. Then he might not mention it again for months, and then he would see something on an angle again somewhere. So, that part has been on and off for years and with no real explanation as to why. I look back on it now and wonder if it is possible that he was starting to have Lewy Body then and that was the only symptoms he was having at the time. If it was, it had taken all of these years to magnify itself to this point now where he has all of these distortions, visions, flashing lights and other symptoms."

Laura answered back, "Wow! I guess we'll never really know for sure."

"That's true," I responded. "John seems to be having the visions of things being tipped more and more all of the time. The flashing lights are increasing, and it makes me wonder how bad it will get for him?"

CHAPTER FIVE

I sat in the Church pew and bowed my head. No one was near me except for John who sat quietly beside me, and I felt at one with God at that moment.

"Please Lord, look after John. Forgive me for getting angry with you because of John getting sick. I believe that there is a reason for everything and you must have a reason for this. Please give me more time with him and let me find a way to help him and maybe help others at the same time. I need you to give me strength Lord, to do what I have to do. Please give me compassion and understanding, and I need you to have compassion on me for being weak. I am making many mistakes, and I am trying to learn one day at a time on how to cope. I put it all in your hands, Lord. Thank You. Amen."

I looked up and saw Adrian, Natalia and the twins, Vince and Alyssa coming into the Church. They had smiles on their faces.

I was nervous as I was about to get my First Communion and Adrian was going to be my sponsor. I had a big fear that somehow I would let him down.

Adrian looked nervous as well. They sat down in the pew next to John and I, and within a few seconds of them getting there, the service began.

Every time I am in the St. Peter's Catholic Church in Trenton I feel at such peace. The world with all of its worries are somewhere outside the doors of this beautiful building, and for a few minutes each time I'm there, I feel that I am in the presence of God.

Father Tim performed the ceremony. He has a fantastic sense of humour, and with a few jokes and smiles, he made sure that everyone was comfortable with what was happening. The service went quickly, and before I knew it, I was standing with Adrian behind me with his hand on my shoulder as I took my oath to God.

I was so proud to have Adrian as my sponsor. It meant so much to me. My faith was getting me through a lot lately. I would find myself talking to God in my mind not necessarily as a prayer, but just as a conversation telling him my fears or worries. I often wondered how people carry on if they did not have faith in God to give them strength. I have always believed that there is a reason for everything. I have this belief has made some hard times in my life a lot easier to accept.

When the service was over, we went back to Adrian and Natalia's house, and he cooked lunch. My sister Laura had come to give her support in my choice of becoming Catholic, and I truly appreciated having her there. We all had a relaxing time sitting and chatting in the back yard while the children played. Soon the afternoon came to an end, and we said our goodbyes and left.

That evening John and I sat in the living room watching TV. He seemed a little tired, and I could see that he was dozing off in his chair. "How about we make it an early night?" I suggested.

"Sounds like a good idea," he replied. "I've had a lot of flashing lights today."

"Well let's try to get some rest, and maybe you won't have so many flashing lights tomorrow," I suggested. Speaking of tomorrow, if it is a nice day I am going to paint some more of those boards that we bought for the bedroom floor. I'll paint them outside on the deck, and then when they're dry, I will bring them in and install them on the floor."

John just smiled at me and then made his way to the washroom.

The next day it was sunny and warm. There was a light breeze blowing, and there was no prediction for rain.

"Perfect weather today to paint those boards," I said while I was preparing his breakfast. "I am going to go and get started after I clean the kitchen."

While John was eating, I made a coffee and then went to get dressed.

A few minutes later I had my painting jeans and long cotton shirt on that I always wore when I had a large painting job going on. I pulled back my long hair and looked in the mirror and said "yuck," as I saw a tired face staring back at me.

I went into the kitchen and picked up the dishes that now sat empty on the island and put them into the soapy dishwater. Then I grabbed the cloth and wiped the counter down.

"Did you want to come out and sit on the deck as I paint? You can keep me company and entertain me while I'm working."

"Yes, I would like that."

"Great," I smiled, and I picked up his coffee and handed him his cane, and we both walked to the kitchen door. I opened it, and I went through first, holding the door for him. I helped him over to the white bench that sat on the deck, and I put his coffee on the small table that sat beside the chair. I waited for a moment to make sure that he was seated comfortably and then I went to work. I picked up the paint can and stir stick and got all my brushes together. After opening the can and giving it a good stir, I sat up five 4x8ft.; board's on the deck sitting side by side to each other. I placed newspaper under each one to prevent any paint from getting onto the floor and then I started painting.

I listened to the birds singing in the trees as I worked. Every once in a while there would be a butterfly cross over the deck on its way into the garden. I could hear children's laughter off in the distance as they played outside taking advantage of the beautiful weather and the fact that they were on summer vacation.

I looked over at John, and I could see that he was enjoying being outside. He had a peaceful look on his face as he sat just sat there.

"Are you enjoying the day?" I asked.

John looked at me and smiled, "It is nice out here. The trees give it a lot of privacy from the road. You don't even know someone is walking down the sidewalk until they get right in front of here."

"It is nice out here," I smiled back. "I hope it doesn't get any hotter. The temperature is perfect for painting. The breeze will help it to dry even faster. Everything should dry in a few hours, and I can maybe move them all into the house by tonight."

About an hour later I was finished painting, so I went into the house and got us both another coffee. I sat on the bench beside him and we both just enjoyed the moment. It was nice not to be rushing off to a Doctor's appointment to get more tests done. It was lovely to sit in the peace and stillness of the afternoon and enjoy the moment together.

John started to say something, "I thought that we…" then his voice drifted off.

I waited a few minutes, and then I said, "You were saying?"

"I don't remember what I was trying to say. That happens a lot lately."

"That's alright," I said trying to sound light-hearted when I could feel my heart sinking.

"You'll remember later, and then you can tell me. Until then how would you like some lunch?"

He smiled, and I stood up and then helped him to his feet. I handed him his cane, and we walked back inside together. After lunch, he sat in his chair, and I turned a movie on for him.

"I see that the wind is starting to pick up. I am going out to pick up a board that has blown over," I said.

John looked up and smiled and then went back to watching his movie. It was a cowboy movie which was his favourite type of entertainment.

As the day went on the wind continued to pick up, and several times I had to go outside and pick up some boards that had gotten blown over. By four O'clock that afternoon the wind was getting strong. I heard a couple of boards blow over again and I thought to myself that I had better go and pick them up before they take off.

I was amazed at how powerful the wind had become. I picked up one board only to have another board blow over. So I rushed over and picked that up and then another one blew over as I tried to sit that one back down again. It was becoming a struggle. As I bent over to get another board, two boards blew over hitting me at the same time and almost knocking me over.

"Wow!" I exclaimed out loud. I had begun to struggle with the boards, and I was now gasping for air as I tried to get out from under the boards.

I tried to push the boards off me, and more began to fall. "Shit," I yelled out in frustration.

I heard a noise at the screen door, and I looked up hoping that John was coming out to help me. Instead, he looked outside at what all the commotion was and saw that it was me. John did not realize the struggle that I was having, and I guess he felt that it was just me out there and no need to worry about anything as I had it under control. So he just closed the door.

Shock and dismay hit me at the same time. I continued to struggle with the boards as they continued to fall on me. How prophetic that he should do that, I thought to myself. It was so symbolic of what was happening in our lives. Things were falling on me that I had to handle and he was not with it enough to help almost like a door closing.

Tears ran down my face as I struggled to put the boards upright again. I crumpled to the floor of the deck and sobbed for about ten minutes. That was the moment that I finally had to accept what was happening in our lives. I couldn't make any more excuses for myself. I had to accept that he was not going to get much better; he was only going to get worse, and I needed to start to prepare for that.

"How do I do this God? What is it that you want me to do?" I asked looking up at the sky. I got up from the floor of the deck and sat on the bench and wiped away any evidence of tears. I could not go inside and let him know that I was upset. I had discovered somewhere along the way that when I get upset then so does John, Then his tremor gets worse, and his memory gets worse. So the best thing for us both was to stay calm and keep him quiet.

There were times when I just wanted to be allowed a few minutes to fall apart and feel sorry for him and me, but that was a luxury that I could not afford.

A few minutes later I went back into the house, and he was sitting watching a movie and acted as if he had no idea that the wind had blown the boards over. I just smiled at him and made my way to the washroom. I closed the door and stood there leaning on it; I felt so empty at this moment. There were a thousand thoughts going through my brain, but not one made any sense to me. I felt tears begin to roll down my face again and I stepped away from the door and leaned on the counter and sobbed.

About five minutes later I knew I had to pull myself together. So I stood up straight and turned the tap on, and got a hand full of water and washed my face. I took a big breath and looked in the mirror and said, to the pale person looking back at me, "I can do this."

I started thinking about some of the things that I had read. A person with Lewy body can change their physical and mental conditions quickly. The way they are one minute is not the way they are the next minute, and as a caregiver, I knew I had to act accordingly. So I needed to learn to accept the surprises be it good or bad. Cherish the good ones and learn from the bad ones. I am having read enough to know that every person with Lewy Body acts differently and I considered us both very lucky that he had not had any episodes of real anger or lashing out. Some people have it a lot worse, and I needed to keep reminding myself of that and be grateful.

I closed my eyes and said softly, "Lord make me strong." I opened the door and stepped out. As I passed John, I asked him, "Can I get you anything?"

He just smiled and turned back to the TV.

I went over to my laptop computer picked it up. Once more I would spend some time researching any Lewy Body information that I could come up with for a while.

As I was getting John ready for bed that night, he sat on the side of the bed and said, "I thought that I had a nail in my boot so I took it off and looked and it turned out that I had five."

I raised my eyebrows and smiled at him as I saw that familiar smirk come on his face let me know that he was only too aware of the fact that he was funny.

I giggled and relished in the moment of having him back with me again.

I wondered to myself about the brain problem and mused that maybe he did not have Lewy Body, but some rare disease that makes the patient not only see things funny but also laugh at many things.

"Don't forget you have a dentist appointment tomorrow," I said as I tried to help him lie down.

It was strange, but for a couple of weeks now, John had been having a problem with trying to find a way to lie down on the bed at night time. It had become a big issue.

He felt like he was going to fall and because of this, it had made him scared of lying down on the bed. I would stand beside him as he would struggle and try and manoeuvre himself onto the bed. I tried each night to raise his legs, but it was almost like he was fighting it. He would not be able to help me, and his legs were massive to me. So I would try and talk him into a sitting position first and then try and talk him into lying down.

"John just lie back on your side and slide your butt into the centre of the bed."

"I can't. I'm trying, but I can't slide over, and I feel like I am falling off the bed," John responded.

"No, you're not falling. I am right here, and you will hit me before you hit the floor. So let's try it again. Try to sit back as far as you can and then let yourself fall over onto your side until your head hits the pillow."

"I can't do it," he said frustrated. "I don't seem to be able to pick up my legs onto the bed."

"Well then let's try raising the head of the bed, and you can just sit back and then I will bring the head of the bed down, and I will help you raise your legs that way," I said. "Remember that was why we bought the adjustable bed so that we can adjust it to the way you need it."

"It's not working," he said again in despair.

"Well let's just take a break for a minute and then we will try again," I suggested as I sat on the bed beside him.

That night we tried for more than an hour to get him lying down. About half an hour later he was up going to the washroom, and then we started all over again. The next time was a little better, and he was back in bed in about twenty minutes.

The next morning as he ate breakfast, he looked over at me and asked, "If your Dentist removes your bicuspid does that mean you are having a gender problem?"

I choked on my coffee!

CHAPTER SIX

In January after John had started having the visions and distortions, I decided that I would do music therapy on him. I had noticed that John was doing something that he had never done before and that was humming a song. In all of the years of knowing him, John had never once sung a song or paid much attention to music at all. I asked him once if he did not like music and he responded that he didn't care one way or the other and because of his hearing aids most music did not sound right to him anyway.

So when he started to hum a tune, it was noticeable to me. I was also fascinated that it was always the same tune. I made a mental note that he seemed to do it if he was feeling uncomfortable about something. John would sometimes start to hum if there were no other distractions, and again always the same tune. At first, I did not want to mention it as I did not want to stop him from doing it. He always seemed to have a look on his face that let me know he was doing it absent-mindedly.

Finally, one day, I was getting him ready to go out, and he was doing it, so I asked him, "So what is the song that you're humming?"

"I didn't know I was humming a song."

"Yes, you do it rather often. I thought maybe it was something that you like."

"I have no idea what it is," he answered rather perplexed. "I had no idea that I do it."

"Well maybe we have a new songwriter on the horizon," I said trying to sound light-hearted about it.

I thought a lot about it afterwards, and I had read somewhere about music therapy. I also had heard the statement, many times, over the years, that music soothed the savage soul. So I began to think that maybe music, in this case, might be a good thing.

So for the next few weeks, I started our days off with music in the morning. I refused to turn on the news or anything else on TV until he had least had had his breakfast and pills. I started with soft, easy listening music that was just instrumental with no words. I noticed in the first couple of days that he seemed more relaxed in the mornings.

So then I started with the instrumental for about an hour and then switched it to the fifties and sixties music for about another hour if we were not going anywhere. That brought back memories, and John would start talking about different things he remembered from a particular song.

Then one afternoon he said to me. "I don't know what is wrong with the TV; it doesn't make any sense to me. No matter what I'm watching, a movie or a commercial, nothing makes any sense any more. I know that I have said that before but what is wrong with the writers of TV and commercials? How do they expect anyone to understand what they are trying to say?"

"Give me a few minutes, and I'll change the channel and try to find something else that you will like, but I need to take the dogs out for a quick pee at the front of the house. I already have them on a leash, and I have put Leo in the backyard already. I'll be back in just a minute." I had been cooking, and the dogs were letting me know that they had waited long enough and they needed to go. "I don't think I can make them wait any longer," I said to John as he sat in his chair looking frustrated at the TV.

"Alright," he said.

As I walked out the front door, I wondered why he was having such a hard time to understand what was on the TV lately. It seemed that he mentioned not understanding the TV a couple of times a week.

I was gone less than four minutes as the two little dogs went on the lawn at the front of the house and then we turned and quickly made our way back inside.

As we stepped through the front door, I took the two small dogs off their leash and went to the living room to change the channel on the TV. Much to my surprise, John was not there.

I looked in the hallway, and the stair lift was still on the main floor letting me know that he had not gone upstairs. Oh No, I thought to myself, and I turned and rushed out the back door and down the steps to the back yard. There was John in the dog pen with Leo.

"John," I called out, "What are you doing?"

"I was looking for Leo. I didn't know where he was. I thought I had better find him because you weren't home."

"I told you I was just taking the two small dogs for a quick pee out on the front lawn," I responded. "I don't want you to come in here without me knowing it. You could fall and get hurt. Or the dog jumps on you because Leo thinks you are going to play with him and knock you down.

"I guess I didn't hear you," he said visibly upset.

"That's fine, I'll take him in now, and we will have some dinner. You come with us. Leo wants to know that you are inside too," with that I called Leo who followed me into the house. We waited inside the door until John came and then we went up the back stairs together."

I made a mental note to myself that I had to make sure that he understood from now on where I was and for how long. I took a big breath and thought to myself that I had to stop taking things for granted and make sure that he always understood what I was doing.

Leo came over to me and leaned up against me and then went over and leaned on John, who had just gone back and sat down in his chair again in the living room.

I walked over and patted, the dogs head and said to him, "You stay with Dad."
I then walked away and back into the kitchen to finish cooking dinner.

He was obedient about being told to stay with John, and he would stand beside him and wait for me to come back before leaving. I thought that was smart of the dog since he was never trained to do that. Something about him seemed to let him know that John needed him near him.

Later that evening I found that exhaustion had set in on me and I was ready for bed around 10 pm. I looked at John who was looking somewhat tired, and I said, "I'm tired and think I would like to go to bed, how about you?"

"Yes I could use some sleep," he responded.

Within an hour the house was dark except for a few night lights that I always left on and the dogs were settled in for the night. John was drifting off to sleep almost as soon as his head hit the pillow. I closed my eyes, and I had fallen into a deep exhausted sleep and did not hear or feel John get up during the night. He had gone to the washroom but was struggling to make it back to bed. I was unaware of that until the dog Leo came to my side of the bed and woke me up. He kept nudging me with his nose until I finally awoke enough to pay attention to him. As soon as I opened my eyes, he ran out of the room. Leo then turned and came back to the door to see if I was following him. Then ran back to John and stayed with John who was in the hallway bent over, until I got there, and then he ran back to the bedroom and laid down on his bed and stayed out of the way until I got John back into the room.

It took about ten minutes to get John back to the bed as it was if his legs did not want to work correctly. He was having a tough time getting one foot in front of the other. When I did finally get him to the bedroom and had him sitting on the side of the bed, he was unable to lie down. It was as if he could not understand how to pick up his legs and slide his body back onto the bed. It was about another twenty minutes of suggesting different ways to lie down.

"I'm going to fall," he stated.

"Trust me you can't fall. If you start to fall you are going to fall into me first as I am right here beside you. I have put this chair beside the bed so that you will bump into it before you start to fall. If you do fall you are going to fall onto me," I said as I tried to raise John's legs onto the bed.

"No, no I am falling," he said alarmed.

"You are not falling. You are sitting on the bed back far enough that you would have to jump forward to try and fall," I said trying to make light of it.

"I can't do it," he repeated.

"John you do it every night. You've been doing it your whole life. You are not going to fall. I won't let you fall, I promise you."

He seemed to relax a bit, and I just waited for a few minutes and said nothing and did nothing and then slowly I raised his legs. He was very stiff, and he did not help, but at least he did not fight it anymore. Finally, his legs where on the bed and I said to him try to lie on your side and get comfortable.

It took about another five minutes, and finally, he was lying down. He did not look comfortable, but at least he was flat on the bed. I covered him up.

I bent down and patted the dog's head, "Wow! You are great. Thank you so very much, Leo." I patted him on the head, and then I went back to bed.

The next day John had an appointment in Trenton, so we stopped over to see Adrian, Natalia and the kids. We sat around their table talking, and the kids wanted to play a game that we have often done, where one person starts a story with a sentence and then the next person says another line, and then the next person says another sentence, and we all take turns at making up a story. We went around the table each person taking a turn at making something up for the story, and when it got to John, the kids said, "Alright Grandpa, it's your turn to make up something to keep the story going."

John sat there at the table looking confused and not saying anything, we all waited a minute or two and then Vince stated as if it was nothing new, "That's alright; Grandpa is not with us right now."

I was so shocked to hear this seven-year-old say that. We had never really discussed with the children about John and what he was experiencing with the illness. They seemed to have an understanding about the Parkinson's, but no one had ever discussed with them about Lewy Body, and I was thrown back to hear him say that as if it was just a way of life. They saw no need to get upset and felt we should carry on. He seemed to know that Grandpa would be back when he was ready.

Later at home, John still seemed a bit out of it, so I put some music on, and we ate dinner listening to the fifties. He seemed to respond to it, and by the end of the meal he was talking and laughing about old times he had when he was young.

That night I suggested we go to bed early again as we both were yawning and acting tired. I got John in bed and went to have a quick bath and by the time I got back he was sound asleep. I said goodnight to the dogs and crawled into bed. Leo came over and checked on me. He had been doing that now for about two months. He would let me get John in bed and say goodnight to him and the other dogs, and he would wait until the lights were out and then come and say goodnight to me. I spoke to everyone that the dog tucks me in.

I smiled, hugged him and said, "Good night Leo. Sleep well."

John was extremely restless most of the night. He had been mostly on my side of the bed tossing back and forth and finally around 4:30 am. John seemed to settle down and lay still. I drifted off, and the next thing I heard was a loud crash and then Leo gave a sharp bark as if trying to call to let me know that something was wrong. John had fallen out of bed. The dog was with him instantly and stayed by his side until I got there and then once again without being told he just went to his bed and laid down getting out of the way immediately.

"Are you alright?" I asked John.

"I'm fine," he said.

"Just take your time, and we will get you up slowly." I directed him. It took a few minutes, and finally, he was up and leaning on the side of the bed. It took another minute or two and then I had him sitting on the bed again."

"Thank God you did not get hurt," I said as I looked him over to see if there were any cuts or bruises, but I could not see anything. "Are you sure you are alright?"

"I think so," he answered.

"Good I'm glad, but you just about gave me a heart attack. My heart is still pounding in my chest. I'm not a big fan of waking up with a bang," I laughed.

Slowly I guided him to lie down. I helped with raising his legs on the bed, and he sunk back into his pillow without much trouble. I was surprised how easy it went compared to the night before. I covered him up and said, "Just try to close your eyes and get some sleep."

"Alright," he answered.

I bent down and talked to Leo for a few minutes. "You are such a good boy for helping. Thank you, Leo." I petted his head as he stretched out as if he was exhausted and closed his eyes. He was asleep before I walked around my side of the bed.

The next morning John was up and eating breakfast as if nothing had happened the night before.

"Are you feeling alright?" I asked as I poured him a coffee.

"I feel fine. Maybe a little stiff from the fall but nothing hurts," he smiled reassuringly. He finished his breakfast and walked out of the kitchen. I could hear him taking the stair lift upstairs. A few seconds later I heard Leo making a noise in the hallway. Not a bark but more of a whine. I left the kitchen and went into the hall to the stairs and noticed that John had taken the stair lift only halfway up and then got off the stairlift and walked up the rest of the way. Leo was alerting me to this.

I ran up the stairs to find that John was in the washroom. I waited at the top of the stairs and said to him as he came out of the bathroom. "John you cannot get off the lift before it reaches the top. That is way too dangerous. You need to stay on until you safely reach the top."

"I can walk faster than that thing can go. It slows me down when I am on a mission," John smiled mischievously.

"Well ride it back down then," I said as I pushed the button to get it to come up the rest of the way to the top of the stairs.

"Alright if it makes you feel better."

"It does. I don't want you to walk on the stairs anymore as you are too unsteady on your feet. You never know when your legs might feel weak and give out on you. The last thing we want is for you to fall."

"Alright, I'll ride that slow thing just for you."

I shook my head smiling and motioned for him to sit down in it as I moved out of his way. I waited at the top of the stairs while he rode it down and then I walked down.

"What would you like for dinner?" I asked trying to change the subject when I got to the first floor where he was standing waiting for me to arrive.

"Room at the table," he chuckled.

I made a face at him and then hugged him.

It was a relief that he had a sense of humour and that it was staying with him no matter what else was happening or how he felt.

Leo had been waiting in the hallway downstairs the entire time and now came over to us and brushed up against my legs. I looked down at him, smiled, patted his head and said, "Leo is the one that told me that you had gotten off the stair lift and walked upstairs."

John smiled at the dog and said, "I told you not to tell. If you are going to snitch on me, then I'm not giving you a treat."

Leo ran and got his ball and tried to hand it to John, "Oh sure try to butter me up now by giving me a treat are you?"

We both laughed as he tossed the ball and Leo went to fetch it.

It was moments like this that made life more relaxed, and I would get the false impression that John was alright and maybe Lewy Body was a misdiagnosis of something else.

A few minutes later John sat at the counter in the kitchen, and I said, "Well how about some pasta for dinner tonight?"

He looked at me, and I could see that things had changed. There was that blank look back in his eyes. I turned so he could not see my face and leaned up against the counter with tears in my eyes. I took a big breath and blinked away the tears. I walked over to where John sat, and I whispered, "Please don't go yet, we were having so much fun."

My heart had sunk into a dark place that it goes when I see him retreat into that dark space in his brain. To me, it is like knowing that he is in a torture chamber where he has no control over what happens next. I have no control over how he is, and I can't stop him from visiting that dark space of emptiness. I enjoy his company so much when he is with it. I miss him so much when he mentally leaves even if it is only for a few minutes.

In one way I was starting to get used to the interludes of emptiness that occurred now almost every day, but at the same time, I was having a hard time accepting the intervals.

John was having fewer visions now that the medications were cut back, but he was still having issues with memory, double vision, and flashing lights.

He said the double vision was coming and going and the flashing lights were happening more and more and meanwhile the distortions of the faces where a bit less than they had been.

I looked at the calendar and saw that tomorrow is the appointment at Sunnybrook Hospital in Toronto to see what the top specialist think they can do if anything for John concerning his eyes and the crater behind the eye.

As I gave John dinner, I said to him, "I looked at the calendar and tomorrow is your appointment that we have been waiting patiently to arrive. We have to get up early tomorrow so that we can leave in plenty of time so that we are not rushing. I hate driving on the 401 highway. I will drive the Trans Canada Highway any day, but the 401 always makes me nervous. Remember the time we were going to Toronto, and we were travelling down the 401 and all of a sudden we had a four or five-foot metal pole swinging and hoping its way down the highway at us? It had come off the back of a truck. It just missed us by a few inches. It narrowly missed some other vehicles on the road as well. Someone was watching over us that day."

John shook his head and said, "Yes I do remember that. It was a scary moment."

The next morning we were up early, and we left the house in plenty of time to make the appointment. I stopped and put gas in the car and then we started down the highway heading to Toronto. John was quiet for a few minutes, and then out of the blue he said, "We are off just like a wooden leg."

"Where do you come up with this stuff?" I laughed.

"I have no idea. It's just stuff that pops into my head," he smiled.

A few hours later we sat in the office of the specialists that we can come to see. The Dr. looked at John and asked, "Tell me, John, what bothers you the most?"

John was slow in replying and then said, "I can't read. I can't see well enough to read anything.

If I take the time to try and read, it takes me so long that when I get to the end of a sentence, I can't remember what the first part of the sentence said. I also have double vision and flashing lights."

The Doctor looked over at me as if I should confirm this, so I shook my head, yes and then said, "John has had distortions since December where he sees people's faces distorted. He may see someone with missing eyes or a mouth where an eye should be, just like cartoon characters. Then about a few months ago he started having what he termed as fish scales on flat surfaces and counter tops, walls etc. about a month after that then he started getting flashing lights. Lately, he has been talking about having double vision."

"So what did his Family Doctor say about all of this?"

"He ordered the MRI and the brain scan, and that is when it was discovered that John has the plaque growing on the brain. From those results and with the symptoms that John has it was determined that he probably has Lewy Body."

"I have the results here and well it is hard to determine Lewy Body. I think John needs to have someone looking after his tremor. Why do they think he has Parkinson's?"

I sighed and said, "Once again it is through the process of elimination and ruling out all other diseases, then they feel that it is the right diagnoses to give John. He had a lot of tests done, and he has seen a Doctor in Kingston, and it is felt that Parkinson is probably what he has."

He checked John over and said, "Well I don't see anything that I can do for you.

There is no damage to the optic nerve, but you do have cataracts, but your eye specialists in Peterborough will look after these for you. I am more concerned with your tremor and who is looking after it for you," the Doctor stated.

I was surprised to hear that. Since the Doctor was an eye specialist's, I was surprised to hear that his concern was a tremor.

"I would like you to see a Doctor at Toronto Western Hospital. He is good with Parkinson like diseases. Would you like me to send you there? Now that you know me you can come back here next year and I can check on your eyes again in a year, but you should go and see this Doctor. I will have him contact you. It will take a lot of time before you see him because these Doctors are very busy, but it will be worth the wait."

I looked over at John who was sitting looking at the Doctor and said, "I want someone to prescribe a pair of glasses so that I can read. Can you do that?"

"Oh no John, glasses will not help you, you need to have your specialist in Peterborough remove those cataracts, but even then glasses won't help you. The hole behind the eye is not operable and maybe removing cataracts will help a bit with your vision but not much."

"So you can't give me glasses to read?" John asked disappointedly.

"No, but I will sit up this appointment for you to see this Doctor at Toronto Western Hospital. He can maybe help you."

"Well, I want to be able to read. I want a prescription for glasses."

The Doctor looked over at me, and I stood up and took a step towards John who was still sitting in the examining chair with a confused look on his face. I handed him his cane and grabbed hold of his arm and started to help him up. I could tell that he was tired and he was having a hard time to grasp the fact that this Doctor would not prescribe glasses.

As we made our way to the parking lot, John stopped walking and asked me, "So what do you think? Is he going to be able to help me?"

I thought to myself that it was not fair that I had to try and somehow make him understand that there was no real help for his eyes. It is so important to him to read again.

"Well John," I said trying to choose my words carefully so that I did not take away hope from him. I truly believe that everyone needs hope to hold onto especially in a difficult situation. "I think we need to see the specialists in Peterborough and see when she is going to remove those cataracts and then we will go from there and see what type of glasses you need."

He seemed to accept that and went quietly into the car. Traffic was heavy, and it took a long time just trying to get away from the Hospital. About twenty minutes later we had cleared the chaos of the Hospital traffic, and now we had to deal with city traffic at rush hour. I made my way to the 401 Highway and managed to get on without much difficulty and then it took about 3.5 hours getting home. It was a long hard drive for John who had become very tired. I felt so bad that it was not a positive trip.

As we neared home, John seemed to perk up a bit and asked again, "So do you think I can get a prescription for glasses to read with from the other Doctor?"

"Well let's see what she has to say when we see her next week. Maybe she will be able to do those cataracts soon, and then things will change for the better for you."

John sat back in his seat and smiled, "Yes I hope so. I miss reading my books."

"I know you do. I think it would be great if you can read again. So let's keep positive thoughts," I smiled over at John as I pulled into the driveway.

The next morning I was doing more research on the computer as we had a few hours before going to the Doctor appointment. I received an e-mail from a Parkinson's foundation in Australia. I had contacted just about everyone, everywhere that might give me more insight. The message in the e-mail contained information about research being done in South Korea where they have discovered that people with early Parkinson's disease have a thinning of their retinas. This is the thin layer of sensitive nerve cells at the back of the eye. I found the information very informative, and I hoped I would learn more about it later when more research information becomes available.

When John got up, I said to him, "How about we go after breakfast and get you some glasses. We can try to find something that might work for you so that you can read."

"Yes, alright," he said.

About an hour later we stood in the dollar store where he tried on one pair of glasses after another and finally decided on one that seemed to allow him to read something printed on a card in the store.

We paid for them and made our way home again where he sat down at the kitchen counter, and I handed him a magazine on tools and the weekly newspaper.

I stood back and watched as he tried to read with the new pair of glasses. "Well, what do you think?"

"It helps a bit. I have a hard time to get what the sentence says as it takes me so long to get to the middle or the end of the sentence, that I can't remember what the beginning of the sentence says," John replied.

"Well maybe just, take your time. Don't rush and it will get a little easier," I said trying to sound encouraging. While deep down inside, I thought that John is just unable to remember the beginning of a sentence, but not because of the eyes, but because of the Lewy Body. It broke my heart because I know how important it is to him to be able to read. That is what he has his heart sit on. He is willing to accept everything else that is happening to him but find a way to help him see better.

CHAPTER SEVEN

Its September now and there seems to be a competition between the last of summer and the beginning of fall. Hot, humid weather prevails on most days. Once in a while, we get a cold day letting us know that fall is on its way. The leaves are just starting to change colour and giving the impression of the colourful beauty that is still to come. The days, for the most part, have been hot and humid. Great for all of the heat lovers but enough is enough for the rest of us who enjoy the crisp, fresh air, instead of the stagnate soupy atmosphere.

It has been unbearable to even sit under a tree in the shade, so John has been inside watching TV a lot. He does better if he is more active, but in this heat, he could not do anything. The Parkinson's has affected his sweat glands so that it makes it hard for him to sweat. Therefore it is essential that he stays as cool as possible.

We are lucky as we have central air and that makes the house our escape from the summertime heat. We love sitting outside under the big maple trees that give off a lot of shade and causing the temperature about ten degrees cooler under them, but this year with the humidity it has made it unbearable to even sit under the trees.

At the moment the house is quiet. It's 2:25 am. and I finally decided to get up. John has been dreaming, and in his sleep, he is restless, and he is kicking out his legs and feet. He managed to get turned over on his stomach and then he started hitting the bed with his hand as if he was trying to push something away from him.

"John, wake up. You need to turn over," I said as I shook him trying to wake him up.

In a muffled voice he replied, "I am turned over."

"You need to lie on your side so that maybe you can be a bit more comfortable."

"I'm on my side," he responded as he lay on his stomach.

There have been a few times over the last few months where I find it impossible to wake him up entirely, and this was going to be one of those times. So rather than stay and run the risk of accidentally getting in the way of his fist while he is sleeping, I decided to come downstairs and sit in my office for a while. I can hear him still if he gets up or needs something as the bedroom is at the top of the stairs and my office is just off the hallway at the bottom of the stairs.

I dusted, straightened up my desk, and filed things away that I have been tossing onto my desk for the last week or so.

It needed to be done, and I never seem to find the time to do it, so I figured now was as good a time as any.

It was too quiet, and I decided to turn on some soft music. I just sat for a long time at my desk and absorbed the music after I finished cleaning. No real thoughts were with me, but after about an hour of peaceful bliss, exhaustion set in and I decided to go back to bed and hopefully get him turned over for the rest of the night, so I can get some sleep as well without having to worry about getting hurt. He would never do anything to hurt me on purpose, but in his sleep, he has no idea what he is doing.

I have read about people with dementia and Lewy Body getting aggravated at night time, and they can become violent. They think that someone is after them or that someone has turned into an evil person. Some people believe that they see ghosts or something that is very upsetting to them. If they feel they are in danger, they are known to act out their dream.

Lewy Body is not like that. John is still sleeping and lying in bed, but doing aggressive tossing and turning more than anything, but once in a while he does lash out as if hitting someone. He is not getting up out of bed and acting out a dream.

A friend asked me once why I don't sleep in one of the other rooms, but if I did, I would fall asleep and not know what is going on. I fear him getting up and getting hurt. So I stay with the thoughts that I will catch up on sleep eventually which usually means that one night out of about four or five, I fall into a deep sleep and don't hear anything unless the dog wakes me up.

This way if he wakes me up because he is having a restless night, then I get up and listen for what is going on, which up to now has only been while he is lying down. He has never gotten aggressive or fear-driven during the night, and I pray he never will.

I turned the lights off in my office about 4 am., and I went back to bed. I was hoping that he would have settled down. I went into the spare room and retrieved a pillow from the bed and put it between us so that should he lash out he would hit the cushion first.

The next morning I said, "Do you remember anything about last night?"

"No not really," he answered thoughtfully as if trying to remember. "I don't feel like I slept very well."

"Well, welcome to the group," I said smiling as I prepared breakfast.

The phone rang, and it was my neighbour and friend Jackie, "I was wondering if you have the time to take me to Peterborough today? I have a few things I have to get done. I always feel so guilty about asking you, but since I don't drive, I have no other way to get there."

"I can take you today, but it will be about an hour as I am doing laundry and I want it to finish before I go and I do not want to leave John alone. He has been feeling a bit unsteady on his feet. The last thing I want to do is have him fall, and I'm not here to help him. It makes it so very difficult since he is not able to dial 911 if he had an emergency because of the tremor."

"Yes I never thought of that fact before, but his tremor would make dialling for help difficult," Jackie said in amazement.

John walked into the kitchen and stood there listening. I watched him as I could tell he heard something, but I had no idea as to what. He finally asked me, "Do you hear a cricket?"

"No," I answered slowly thinking about what he might be hearing, and then I realized what it was, "That is just the washing machine."

"Wow! You wouldn't think that they would last long in there would you?"

I raised my eyebrows at him.

That old familiar smirk crossed his face, and he smiled and walked away.

About an hour later we were standing in the parking lot of Home Depot in Peterborough.

"Oh look out," cried out Jackie pointing to John who was behind me.

I turned quickly, and I saw him trying to gain his composure. He looked like someone doing ballet in the parking lot.

He looked at us both and gave a mischievous smile. "What I am just trying out some new dance steps," he exclaimed.

"Just be careful I don't want to pick you up off the ground," I stated, as I stepped towards him and took hold of his arm.

Jackie exclaimed, "Wow John you scared me. I thought you were falling."

"Listen, Jackie; we don't need anything in the store, so we're just going to go and check out the garden centre while you go do what you need to. We'll meet you back here at the car when you are finished shopping," I said as I guided John towards the sidewalk.

"Yaw, that sounds good. I won't be long," Jackie said as she took off towards the store entrance.

John and I strolled towards the garden section of the store. We took our time going up and down a few isles of flowers and plants — bushes and trees where planted in containers standing to the sides of the centre.

"Do you want to go inside," I asked looking at John.

"Sure let's check it out," he said as he moved towards the door that led into the store.

Inside they were sitting up for Halloween. There were costumes hanging and new Halloween statues that were life-sized and lights flashing, with music playing.

"Wow!" I exclaimed, as we took a few steps inside and looked around. "There is a lot of stuff to scare the little ones."

John started to point to something that had caught his interest, and suddenly he was swaying and just about to fall over. I grabbed his arm and tried to steady him.

"Are you alright?"

"I think so, I just turned my head too fast," he said.

"Well, we've seen enough. How about we go back outside and sit in the car.

He shook his head, yes, and we started to make our way to the exit door. He seemed to get more unsteady with every step he took. I saw a bench not far away and said how about we sit on that bench for a few minutes. There were already two people sitting there

But I was sure that John was not going to make it back to the car. As we approached the bench, the man stood up, and the woman slid over making way for him to sit down. They seemed to know he was suffering at that moment.

"Thank you," I smiled at them both.

"No worries," the man said as he stood beside the bench.

I helped John sit down and then I stood beside him while he rested. He seemed exhausted, and I felt that just letting him rest for a few minutes would be best.

"Do you want to wait here while I go and get the car?"

"No, I'll come with you," he said as he struggled to get up.

I helped him up and said, "Stand still for a minute while you get grounded and then we will make our way to the car. It's not far." I said as I pointed to it parked in a handicapped zone.

Within a couple of minutes, I was guiding him back to the car. I assisted him to the passenger side and got him safely seated, and then I went around the driver's side of the vehicle. Jackie came out of the store a couple of minutes later and loaded her parcels in the back of the car.

When we got home, I dropped Jackie at her house and then helped John inside. He seemed very tired, so I got him seated in his chair. I turned the TV on for him and went to get him a decaf coffee. When I returned a few minutes later, he was already sound asleep. I sat his hot drink on the table beside him and stood and watched him. He looked so peaceful, the tremor stopped and his body at complete rest, "I wish you could be like that all of the time," I whispered.

The next morning as we prepared for the day, John was in the kitchen and went to walk around the island, and he suddenly stopped and said, "As I took that step I felt like I was walking into a large black hole."

"What do you mean?"

"I just felt like I was stepping into a massive black hole. I can't explain it better than that."

I was shocked. I had been standing right there. I noticed that John seemed to get unsteady on his feet, but he had to be like that for a few days now, but John had never mentioned anything like this before.

Later that same day, we were back at the Chiropractor's office. As John lay on the table, I said to Dr Cocek, "John has been very unsteady on his feet since the weekend."

John piped up at that moment and said, "My neck hurts."

"Well alright," The Doctor said, "I think it could be due to the stiff neck."

Within a couple of minutes, he had treated John and gave extra attention to his neck area.

As we walked out of the building, John said, "My neck feels a bit better. I think coming here and doing this might be working a bit."

"I know it's working for you. You always stand a little straighter for a few days after being here. Think about it, John. It took you seventy-two years to get to this point with your back, neck and other problems. It will take some patience and time to get it fixed. You have lucked out again, as Dr Cocek is good at his job."

The next day John had another eye appointment with his eye specialist in Peterborough. Her assistant came out and called John into the inner office where she had him sit in a chair.

John sat down, and I sat beside the desk while she called up his chart on the computer.

"Well, John has there been any changes since you were last here?"

"I was at Sunnybrook last week and saw that Doctor who couldn't help me."

"Well let's get you looked at today and see what we can do for you."

John just looked confused at this point, so I piped up and said, "He is the eye specialists that the eye Doctor in Oshawa sent us to, to get another opinion. He said that there was no damage to the eye nerve and that he could not do anything for John."

The assistant looked at his chart and said, "there is no paperwork concerning the visit as of yet. Has there been any change with his eyes since he was here last?"

"He is still getting the flashing lights, and he is now experiencing double vision," I explained.

"Alright John, I want you to read the eye chart for me," she said.

"Do you mind covering his eye," she asked directing the question to me, "As it might be easier if you do it because of the tremor?"

"Sure," I said as I got up and went over to stand beside John. I cupped my hand over his right eye first, and he tried to read the chart. He had a hard time with the letters, and each time he tried to read a line, he would struggle with it."

After a few minutes, the assistant said, "Alright John let's try the other eye."

I went around to the other side of the chair and cupped my hand over his left eye.

Again he attempted to read the chart with difficulty. He hesitated after the third line, and the assistant said, "Keep going, you're on a roll now."

"That's alright someone will catch me," John replied.

We all laughed and then he tried a couple more times and then said, "No that's it, I can't do it."

A few minutes later we saw the Ophthalmologist. She read over the chart and what the assistant had written and then put drops in his eyes so she could check them more closely. "No, your cataracts have not matured enough yet to be able to do the operation. So we will have to wait for another six months."

My heart sank as I knew that was not what John wanted to hear.

John was listening and asked, "Can you write me a prescription for glasses so that I can see to read?"

"When was the last time you had your eyes checked?"

"It was last December," I answered as I knew John would not remember the date.

"Well, then you will have to wait until December, and they might give you a new prescription, but I don't know if it will work. I see here that you have had double vision and I think you need to see your family Doctor about that. When are you seeing him again?"

"He has an appointment tomorrow with him," I responded.

"Well, talk to him about the double vision, and I will see you back here again in about six months. Maybe by then, we can operate on your eyes to remove the cataracts."

Disappointed John and I walked out of the office and onto the elevator. "So does that mean she is not going to prescribe new glasses for me? Why is it so hard for someone to do that? I want to be able to read."

"I know," I responded trying to think of what to say. I walked over to the machine to pay for the parking. I inserted the parking ticket and money into the machine, and while we waited for it to print out, I said to John, "Well how about we go to a dollar store somewhere and see what we can find to magnify the words for you so that maybe you can read."

"Do you think it would work?" He asked.

"Well, we have nothing to lose so let's try and see."

"I just want to go home," he said in despair. "I need something to eat, and I want to relax. I'm tired."

When we got home, he sat in the kitchen and looked completely heartbroken. He accepted a coffee when I offered it to him, and he just took one sip and then it sat there. He sat there just staring into space and not saying anything.

Finally, I asked him, "How about some dinner? Are you getting hungry?"

"I guess so," he responded and then went back to staring into space.

I prepared dinner, and as it was cooking, I was at the kitchen sink with my back to John when I heard him say, "I can't see me."

"What?" I questioned as I turned around to look at him. He had gotten up from the counter and was now standing in front of the kitchen window.

"I don't see my reflection in the window, but yet I can see yours as you walk by."

I walked over beside him and looked into the dark window, and I said, "I can see you. You are right beside me."

He stood there for a minute a bit unsteady on his feet looking into the window and then said, "Well as long as you can see me then I guess I'm in there too."

With my heart in my throat and trying really hard to sound calm I said, "Well how about a nice bowl of ice cream before dinner?" I just wanted to get him away from the window and get his mind on something else.

"Sounds good," he said as he smiled and then turned around and sauntered over to the island and sat down.

The next day we saw Dr Read. We explained to him what happened at Sunnybrook and in the Ophthalmologist in Peterborough with his eyes and how disappointed John was that no one would write a prescribe glasses, because that was all he wanted.

"Well, John you seem to be doing well with cutting back on your Parkinson's medications so if you want we will try to take you off now. How about we do it slowly again just like we have been and we will have you take a pill just at bedtime every other day, and we will see how you do with that," smiled Dr Read.

"Yes that sounds fine," said John as he nodded in agreement.

"Do you have any other questions or concerns, John?"

"Not really," smiled John.

"I just thought you should be aware of the fact that he is a bit more unsteady on his feet the last few days and he still has the flashing lights and double vision."

"How often are you getting that?"

"A few times a day, I think. I'm not sure, but I think so." John replied.

Dr Read looked at John and asked, "How are you feeling otherwise?"

"I feel fine really. There is no pain. A slight headache once in a while but not too bad and I sleep better than I used to," John answered slowly.

"Well, if you have any concerns call me, but otherwise I will see you again in about six weeks," Dr Read said. "I want to watch you walk up the hallway before you leave. Your walking had improved the last time you were here, and I want to see how it is today."

"Alright," John said as he handed me his cane and off he walked down the small hallway of the clinic.

Dr Read stood in the doorway and watched him intently taking in, his gait and stride.

"Alright then, that looks good John," Dr Read smiled.

John held out his hand to the Doctor and said, "Thank You," as they shook hands.

Later that evening John was sitting in his chair watching a movie on TV, and I was in my office and sitting at my desk when suddenly the hydro went off. The house was in total darkness. I got up from my desk and tried to make my way to the office door by feeling for things to help guide me. I went into the living room and said to John, "Stay where you are. Don't get up until I find some candles that I left on the fireplace in the kitchen."

John said to me just as I was passing him, "Do you know what I just discovered?"

"No," I replied, "What is it?"

"I just discovered that the light is not too bright when the hydro goes off."

I smiled and asked him, "Can't you say that with a straight face?"

"How do you know in this darkness that I don't have a straight face?"

"I know you," I replied as I continued onto the kitchen.

CHAPTER EIGHT

"Do you hear that? It sounds like someone drilling something. I can even feel the floor vibrate," stated Adrian as he sat across from John at his dining room table.

"I don't hear anything," said John slowly.

I was in the kitchen washing dishes listening to the noise as well.

"There it is again," said Adrian as he stood up.

"Yes, I heard it too," I responded.

"I can't say I heard anything," said John.

Adrian took a few steps away from the table and then stood still as the sound came again. "I wonder if they are doing some work next door."

I turned off the running water in the sink in the kitchen and stood still and listened. "Can you call your neighbours and ask?"

"I'm going to go down to the basement first and check the furnace," said Adrian as he walked towards the basement stairs that are located off the kitchen.

I stood beside the sink and listened. Again I heard the sound, and I also felt the floor vibrate while Adrian was in the basement.

Adrian made his way back from the basement exclaimed, "There it is again. It's not the furnace as the furnace is not even running at this point."

I took a few steps from the kitchen into the hallway. Again we all heard the unexplained sound. Adrian walked past me into the hallway and made his way over to a thermostat on the wall and looked at it and said, "Everything seems fine with the furnace. When I was down in the basement, I could hear the sound up in the ceiling. I could still feel the vibrations on the floor. It sounds like someone drilling into concrete."

"Yes, I agree that is what it sounds like," I said.

We turned and walked back into the dining room where John was still seated at the table. Adrian sat back down at the table and listened intently as the sound happened again.

"I have no idea what it could be," stated Adrian mystified. "There's the noise and the vibrations again."

"Wow, it is strange," said John shaking his head.

I turned and left the dining room and said on my way out, "I have to go to the bathroom." As I walked away, I heard the sound again and felt the vibrations on the floor. I heard Adrian exclaim, "I wish I knew what it was."

"Yes it is disturbing," stated John.

I returned to the dining room a few minutes later and said to Adrian, "Maybe you should call your neighbour's to see if they are doing some work. It will ease your mind to know it is them working on a project and not something wrong here in your house."

Adrian looked at me with a big smile on his face and said, "It's alright we figured it out."

I was amazed and questioned them both, "So what is it?"

"Go ahead and show her John," said Adrian chuckling.

John smiled and began to swivel in his chair slowly.

Adrian laughed and said, "The bearings have been damaged on that stool. Remember when John sat on this stool about six months ago and it fell over breaking a bearing in the seat? We have never replaced the bearing on the stool, so with John being over six feet tall and his weight just over two hundred pounds, it was creating a grinding noise that no one else sitting on it has managed to make before."

I laughed and said, "Really?

Adrian continued, "So, here we are all trying to figure out the noise, and John swivels on the stool as he is trying to listen to the sounds we are all hearing and saying, "I don't hear anything.""

We all laughed, as John swivelled on the stool again, as he giggled.

"Good going John," Adrian said jokingly. "You broke the bearings before so that you could come back six months later after we had all forgotten about it and play this trick on me. I know what you are up too."

John broke out into laughter.

Adrian and John are like father and son. They are so much alike that Natalia and I are often amazed at how similar they are in their likes and dislikes and the way they approach things. They also love to play little jokes on each other. They both knew that they could rely on each other to always be there if they needed something. So because they are so comfortable with each other, Adrian was not about to let this go unnoticed.

It was nice to see John laughing and smiling. He had a rough start to the day. I helped him get dressed as we had another appointment with his chiropractor. I felt it was essential to keep these appointments, even if he was not feeling well, as it was helping with his stance and also it had helped him on a few occasions with dizzy spells he was having. When we went to leave the house, I just happened to look down at his feet as he was walking out the door and I was shocked to see he had removed everything from his feet and was about to step out into the freshly fallen snow with no shoes or boots on.

"John where are your socks and boots?"

"I left them upstairs," he replied casually.

"You have to have your socks and your boots on. There is snow on the ground outside."

"Alright," he replied and went off to get them.

That evening as John was getting ready for bed he smiled and said, "That was funny at Adrian's today."

I laughed and said, "Yes, but remember what they say about paybacks."

John laughed as I helped him crawl into bed. I pulled the covers up over him as he lay down. He was still smiling as I turned out the lights.

The next morning after breakfast, I walked into the living room and saw the distress on John's face. He was standing near the fireplace, and he had the remote to the TV in his hand, but he was not capable of pushing the button to change the channel.

He was pacing three steps right and then turning and walking two or three feet to the left, in front of the TV. His face was pale, and he seemed a bit disoriented. His tremor had gotten extremely worse, and he acted as if he did not know what to do next.

I walked over to him and put my hand out for the remote. He had a hard time to hand it to me. I instantly put soft music on so that maybe it would help to calm him down.

Every year on this day he gets upset. The eleventh day, of the eleventh month and the eleventh hour are always something that is emotional to him and many others.

Today we had stayed home instead of going out to a Remembrance Ceremony. I had offered to take him to the Trenton Air Base where he had been stationed, but he had declined to say that he did not feel up to it.

John has been complaining the last couple of days that he has a bit of a headache and just not feeling right but not sick, so instead of going to a Remembrance ceremony I turned the TV on, and he sat quietly watching the services on the screen.

I stayed close by, and I noticed a few tears welling up in his eyes and one slide down his cheek that he quickly brushed it away. When the ceremonies where over I had gotten up and went into the kitchen to get him a coffee. When I entered the living room again, I found him with the Parkinson's tremor out of control.

I helped him back to his chair and got him seated, and then I went back into the kitchen and quickly made a sandwich and took it to him. He struggled to get it to his mouth concentrating on his every movement to try and eat without dropping the food on the floor. At this point, his arms, hands, legs and head are all moving out of control.

I sat down near him and started talking about how the dogs were enjoying the cold and the snow. I just wanted to make him start thinking about something else, other than how badly he was feeling at that moment. It seemed to work, and within fifteen or twenty minutes he was starting to calm down and look a bit better. The tremor began to get under control.

John looked at me and said, "It does not take much to get everything out of control."

"Well, it's understandable. These ceremonies are very emotional. It's over now, and you are feeling better," I smiled reassuringly. "How would you like some fresh air? I need to go and get a few things at the grocery store?"

"Yes alright, that might do me some good."

I helped him get his favourite heavy sweater on as it says "We will remember them," on the back. Then I handed him his cane. We made our way out the back door to the car under the carport. I opened the door and said to him smiling, "Your chariot awaits."

He laughed and struggled a bit to get his feet going in the right direction, so he was not tripping over them as he was getting into the vehicle.

I helped him with his seat belt, and then I went around and crawled in the driver's seat and drove off. When we got to the store, I helped him out of the car and gave him a shopping cart and said, "Here it's your turn to drive now. Put your cane in the cart as it will make it easier."

He smiled and took the cart.

I picked up a few things and placed them in the cart as he kept strolling. I stood still and looked at him and smiled.

He looked back at me and gave me his famous mischievous smile and then he asked, "What?"

"Do you remember what it was that I said I had to remember to get when we were out shopping?"

"Yes you said that we needed milk and cheese," he replied.

"Wow! Look at you. You don't have a problem with your memory. I do." I exclaimed, giggling. "I could remember most of the things, but I knew I forgot something."

John just smiled and said without hesitation, "Memory is like fishing, sometimes you have to wait awhile."

I laughed and said, "I think you are right about that. You're quick on the ball with your one-liners."

"Truthfully I never know what is going to come out of my mouth next. I surprise myself sometimes."

"Trust me, you surprise me too," I laughed.

We finished shopping, and we made our way to the car. I put the groceries in the car and got John safely buckled in.

On our drive home I said, "I think I am going to start bringing out the Christmas decorations and maybe put some around the house tomorrow if it is still a nice day." I did not get a response, and I looked over and saw that blank stare on his face.

I sighed, and turned the car into the driveway. I parked, and got out. I went around and opened the door for John. He looked at me for a moment, and then slowly struggled to get out of the car. He stood up but seemed unsteady on his feet. I leaned into the car, grabbed his cane, and handed it to him.

I helped him to the door of the house, and he stood and watched me as I went back to the car and got the groceries out and made my way back to the door.

"Go on in," I said as I nodded my head towards the door. My hands where full with the bags of groceries and I could not move ahead through the door unless he moved first.

I could see the confusion on his face, so I put the groceries down on the ground and just took hold of his arm and guided him through the door and up the back stairs and into the kitchen. I helped him get his sweater off, and I had him sit down in the living room while I went back outside to get the bags of food.

When I got back inside John was standing in the kitchen and talking to Leo. I looked at him and saw that he was back again.

It was moments like this that I just wanted to say to him, "Welcome back," but I never do as I don't think he realizes he was ever gone.

As I put the groceries away, John and Leo left the kitchen and went into the living room. I could hear him talking to Leo, and every once in a while I listened to the ball hit the floor as John tossed it to the dog. Leo was now entertaining John with his toy which is a good thing as it helps to keep John agile for the most part. John is using his arm and hand mussels and joints to toss the ball and then take the toy from the dog when he brings it back.

When I finished putting the groceries away, I walked into the living room to see how things were going.

Much to my surprise, I found John and the dog both down on the ground looking under one of the leather sofas together. I stood there for a moment and watched them. The dog was kneeling so that his front paws were rested on the floor while his back legs were still straight up in the air and his tail was waging quickly from side to side in the excitement of the moment. Leo was thrilled to have John's full attention on his favourite toy. John was in the same stance with his arms bent on the floor, and he had his butt was also up in the air.

"Well this makes a nice picture," I said jokingly.

They both startled at the same time and turned to look at me; both Leo and John had the same look of, Help, on their faces.

I laughed and asked, "Have you two taken up praying?"

"We are praying for some help. We don't seem to be able to reach the ball," said John.

"Well I'll give away my secret to success in these types of matters if you two promise that you won't tell anyone," I said smiling.

"I'm positive that you can rely on me not to tell anyone, but I'm not sure if Leo can keep a secret," John said laughing.

"Well, may I borrow your cane for a moment?"

John handed me the cane and then waited with Leo by his side as they watched me now get down on my hands and knees and move the walking stick under the sofa bringing the ball out with it.

Leo jumped up, grabbed the ball, and then went to sit beside John's chair with the ball in his mouth waiting for John.

I got up, and I helped John to his feet. He made his way back to his chair, and they began to play ball again. John sat in his chair and tossed the ball while Leo retrieved it and then giving it to John to throw it back.

About an hour later John was dosing in his chair, and Leo laid at his feet sound asleep. I hated to wake him up, but I was trying to keep him on a schedule as much as possible. I put my hand on John's shoulder and said, "Dinner is ready."

As we sat at the island in the kitchen, John asked me, "What was that course that you took a couple of days ago on the internet?"

"Oh," I exclaimed as I was surprised that he remembered that I had taken a course. It was a four-week course, but I wanted to finish it in one day, as I was not sure when I would get the time to get back to it again. "It was about Dementia and the arts. Helping people to explore challenge and shape their perceptions of dementia through science and the creative arts."

"Did you complete it all in one day?"

"Yes, I got it done and received my papers already for doing the course."

"Was it interesting?"

"Yes, actually it was. I learned a lot.

It talked about music therapy and how dance therapy can be a good thing for people with Parkinson's, Alzheimer's and Dementia. Moving with the music helps to move the mussels and joints. The benefits of doing creative art such as making things, painting, sketching etc., is using a different part of the brain.

Then there was a section on feeling textures as sometimes a texture will bring back a wonderful memory; maybe from someone's childhood or something that makes them feel good. The course was teaching how Art Therapy can enhance the quality of life for Alzheimer's and Dementia patients."

"I'm glad you enjoyed it?"

"Yes, I did. It talked about how some patients were able to express themselves through art when they were having difficulty letting anyone know how they felt. It gave them a new way to express themselves and communicate with others. It also helped others restore and preserve their sense of self-worth."

John smiled, and said, "I think that's great that you did it."

"Thanks, I'm glad I did it too."

"One part of the course talked about how a man with dementia started painting and how his pictures changed over time as his disease progressed. It became part of a learning tool for Doctors to see the progression of the disease from the paintings the man did."

We finished dinner, and after I had cleaned the kitchen, I said to John, "It's softly snowing outside.

There is no wind to speak of, and it feels enjoyable outside. How about putting your coat on and standing outside while I walk the dogs? You can wait on the deck of the house while I take them to pee, to get some fresh air and enjoy the evening."

"If you want to," he answered smiling.

A few minutes later John watched us from the deck of the house as I paraded the dogs around letting them look for that particular spot to leave their mark on the freshly fallen snow so that all of the other dogs in the area will know that they are still around.

When they finished we walked up onto the deck, and I stood beside John, and we leaned on the railing and just basked in the silence of the evening. No one was around; there were no cars on the road. There was a gentle breeze that felt like it awakened all of the senses. The world had such a clean, crisp feeling to it at that moment, and everything was looking like a winter wonderland postcard.

"I can't believe that it is almost Christmas. This year went so fast," I said. "A lot has happened in this past year."

John nodded in agreement but not saying anything. He was so completely relaxed and enjoying the peaceful moment of the season.

I looked up at the street lights that helped to make the snow even more apparent, and I said to John, "I like watching the flakes of snow swirling and dancing in the street lights. Then softly drifting onto the ground makes the sidewalk and street look like a thousand stars have fallen from the sky.

It looks as if they have gently landed here waiting for someone to come and make a wish."

John looked at me and smiled and asked: "What would you wish for?"

"A million more evenings like this with you."

John smiled and bent down and kissed me and said, "So would I."

FACTS ABOUT DEMENTIA

5% is the percentage of the Canadian Institutes of Health Research's budget invested in dementia says the Alzheimer's Society Canada.

56,000 and rising is the estimated number of Canadians with dementia being cared for in Hospitals even though this is not an ideal location for care.

564,000 Canadians are currently living with dementia.

937,000 is the number of Canadians who will be living with the disease in 15 years.

1.1 Million is the number of Canadians affected directly or indirectly by the disease.

10.4 Billion is the annual cost to Canadians to care for those living with dementia.

25,000 is the number of new cases of dementia diagnosed every year.

16,000 is the number of Canadians under the age of 65 living with dementia.

It is estimated that there are over 400 different types of dementia, the most common of which are Alzheimer's disease and vascular dementia.

Alzheimer's research in the UK estimates that it is possible to have more than one type of dementia at the same time.

It is estimated that for every 100 people with dementia, around 10-15 of them will have DLB.

On a Government of Canada website, it states that according to the World Health Organization that 47.5 million people live with dementia, including Alzheimer's worldwide. By 2031 it is estimated that the total health care costs for Canadians with dementia will have doubled from just two decades earlier, $8.3 billion to $16.6 billion. According to the most recent data available more than 402,000 seniors (65 years and older) are living with dementia in Canada, (excluding Saskatchewan, I'm not sure why). About two-thirds of people living with this disease are women.

FACTS ABOUT PARKINSON'S

Parkinson's disease is named after a British surgeon James Parkinson, who in 1817 wrote an essay on the Shaking Palsy. He is considered the first to observe and describe the symptoms.

It was a French neurologist who later named it the disease Parkinson's.

Symptoms are often on one side more than the other.

Speech can be hindered by a soft voice or decreased articulation, loss of regular inflexion, monotone speech, inflexion and a decrease in facial expressions.

In some people, the decline from Parkinson's may decline slowly and in some cases never lead to significant impairment.

While it is recognized that depression, apathy, and anxiety can be partnered with Parkinson's, it is not uncommon that some people find inspiring and new meaning in their lives after their diagnosis.

Loss of the sense of smell may be one of the earliest symptoms sometimes preceding the onset of the disease that can strike many years later.

Exposure to paraquat a pesticide triples a person's risk of getting Parkinson's disease.

A person has a higher chance of getting Parkinson's if there is a family history of this disease.

STRANGE FACTS

Strangely there is a study that shows that hair colour plays a role. Black hair has less chance of getting dementia, and blond or redheads have a more significant opportunity. Dyed hair doesn't count.

Red hair is made from the L-Dopa, just as dopamine, the substance whose deficiency causes Parkinson's disease.

The Amish community seems to be at higher risk of Parkinson's Dementia than other communities, and some think it is because of the pesticides used in farming.

Trauma to the head and if there is damage done to the cells that produce dopamine, is believed that this can cause Parkinson's Dementia.

Manganese a known cause of Parkinson's if the concentrations are high enough.

Ethnicity studies have shown that Caucasians have higher odds than African Americans.

Illicit drugs may be a factor as the drugs have a bull's eye effect for the dopamine-producing neurons in the brain.

Studies have shown that Parkinson's disease is much more prevalent amongst welders and occupations that are under stress for long periods such as Doctors, Dentists, Teachers, Lawyers, Scientists and more, while the same study shows that creative people and artists are less likely to get Parkinson's disease. It is believed that stress can be a significant factor in this terrible disease.

Many people in the Pacific Island of Guam have developed Parkinson's disease, due to feasting on flying foxes, a species of bat that can be as big as six feet across. This is because bats eat cycad seeds which contain a potent neurotoxin.

In 1875, Henry Huchard had a patient that had all of the symptoms of Parkinson's disease. The patient was only three years old.

As you get older, you have a higher chance of getting Parkinson's disease. Surprisingly enough, Parkinson's is virtually unknown to anyone aged 110 and 120.

Although L-dopa is commonly used to raise L-dopa levels, no other common substance reduces the body's own ability to produce more than L-dopa itself.

Yahya Ibn Sarafyun, a physician in medieval Damascus, devised a formulation for treating symptoms of Parkinson's disease that included frankincense, myrrh and frogs.

Japan is the only country that has more women than men with Parkinson's disease.

L-dopa in seed form was being used in India to treat the symptoms of Parkinson's disease over 6000 years ago.

Although it is widely claimed that there is a massive loss of brain cells involved in Parkinson's disease, not a single piece of research has ever shown this.

For some reason, Bulgarian Gypsies appear to be almost immune to developing Parkinson's disease. All other Bulgarians are ten times more likely to get it.

A new case of dementia is diagnosed about every 3 seconds.

It is estimated that between now and 2050, it is likely that the most substantial rate of increase in dementia will take place in low-income countries and regions including China, India and their south Asian and western Pacific neighbours, making dementia a truly global problem.

NATIONAL RESOURCES & CRISIS HOTLINES

Anxiety Panic Support:

Bell Let's Talk

Canadian Association for Suicide Prevention
204-784-4073

Canadian Mental Health Association
613-745-7750

Collateral Damage
807-768-5217
Toll-Free: **888-835-9041**

Mental Health Commission
613-683-3755

Mood Disorders Society of Canada
519-824-5565

Schizophrenia Society of Canada
1-800-263-5545

Your Life Counts
289-820-5777

Your Life Counts - Military Directorate
In Canada Call
1-800-268-7708
For Veterans, Former RCMP members, their families and Care Givers

British Columbia Resources

Canadian Wellness Program
604-875-6601

Canadian Mental Health Association-British Columbia Division
604-688-3234

Counselling B.C.
Here to Help
1-800-661-2121

Alberta Resources

Canadian Mental Health Association – Alberta Division
780-482-6576

Centre for Suicide Prevention
403-245-3900

Suicide Information and Education Services
403-342-4966

Saskatchewan Crisis Hotline

Saskatoon Crisis Intervention Service
306-933-6200

Mobile Crisis Services
306-757-0127

Saskatchewan Resources

Canadian Mental Health Association – Saskatchewan Divison.
1-800-461-5483

Manitoba Crisis Hotline

Manitoba Suicide Line
1-877-435-7170

Manitoba Resources

Canadian Mental Health Association – Manitoba Division
204-982-6100

Clinic Community Health
204-784-4090

Mental Health Education Resource Centre of Manitoba
1-855-942-6568

Yukon Resources

Yukon Health and Social Services
1-800-667-8346

Mood Disorders Society of Canada – Yukon Division
867-667-8346

Depression Understood
403-668-9111

Nunavut Crisis Hotlines

Nunavut Kamatsiaqtut Help Line
1-800-265-3333

Ontario Crisis Hotlines

Gerstein Crisis Centre
416-929-5200

Ontario Mental Health Helpline
1-866-531-2600

Ontario Resources

Canadian Mental Health Association – Ontario Division
416-977-5580

Connex Ontario Health Services
1-800-531-2600

Crisis Line
In Ottawa: **613-722-6914**
Outside Ottawa: **1-866-996-0991**

Distress and Crisis Ontario
416-486-2242

Family Association for Mental Health Everything (FAME)
416-207-5032

Hincks – Dellcrest Centre
1-855-944-4673

Ontario Association for Suicide Prevention
647-525-6277

Ontario Shores Centre for Mental Health Services
1-800-341-6323

Self – Help Resources Centre
1-866-283-8806

Toronto Distress Centre
416-597-8808

Waterloo Region Suicide Prevention Council
844-437-3247

York Support Services Network
1-866-695-0070

Quebec Crisis Hotlines

Centre de Prevention du Suicide de Quebec
1-866-277-3553

Quebec Resources

Action on Mental Illness
1-877-303-0264

Centre de Prevention de Suicide de Haut-Richelieu
450-348-6300

Movement Sante Mentale Quebec
514-849-3291

New Brunswick Crisis Hotlines

Chimo Helpline
1-800-667-5005

New Brunswick Resources

Canadian Mental Health Association – New Brunswick Division
506-455-5231

Nova Scotia Resources

Canadian Mental Health Association – Nova Scotia Division
1-888-429-8167

Mental Health Foundation of Nova Scotia
902-464-6000

Prince Edward Island Crisis Hotlines

The Island Helpline
1-800-218-2885

Prince Edward Island Resources

Canadian Mental Health Association – Prince Edward Island Division
902-566-3034

Newfoundland and Labrador Resources

Canadian Mental Health Association – Newfoundland and Labrador Division
1-877-753-8550

HELP IS OUT THERE

If you are unable to think of a solution to your problems other than suicide, it is not because other solutions don't exist; it is that you are currently unable to see them at this time. Seek help from a professional, family member, or friend. Every problem has a solution.

Don't feel ashamed or embarrassed to pick up the phone and seek help.

Also, suicide survivors need support for what they are going through. Despair can suddenly become the most significant part of your life while you try to understand and cope with the loss. Remember that it is how someone lived, not how they died that defines someone's life.

Seek support from professionals and friends. Don't let anyone tell you that you are not grieving correctly. There are no right or wrong answers, go with how you feel and allow yourself the time to grieve and heal.

A MESSAGE FOR YOU (CAREGIVERS & FAMILY)

I am not an expert. I have only learned by day to day experiences.

These are just some of the things that I have discovered that has helped me and may work for you.

I know that a positive attitude is essential. Your body language can reveal so much sometimes more strongly than your actual words. The sound of your voice and facial expression can express what you are feeling. It is essential to show that you are comfortable with what is happening at that moment, even if you are not, still give the appearance of confidence and acceptance.

If the person should say something that sounds farfetched and left field, that's alright. Don't argue. Just acknowledge the statement and change the subject.

Try to keep your surroundings peaceful. If the person should get agitated or upset about something, move to quiet surroundings. Make sure that you get their attention. Address them by name and a soft touch on the hand or arm.

Don't stand over them if they are seated, bend down so that you are eye level and speak softly and encouragingly.

Speak slowly in a reassuring voice and use simple words and sentence and if the person is still confused wait a few minutes and then rephrase the question.

Never ask a lot of questions at once. Ask only one at a time that yes or no answers can be given.

If everything seems to be getting out of control, because they have become agitated about something, then redirect and distract their attention, offering something to eat and drink.

It is normal for someone with Alzheimer's or Dementia to feel unsure about themselves. Sometimes they can get perplexed and speak about something that did not occur.

Avoid convincing them that they are wrong and instead, respond with a warm smile and change the subject.

Keep activities, to one at a time. Don't overload them by telling them that you are going to do several different things. Instead, help them get through one activity and then slowly move onto something else. Never rush anything or make them feel that they are being rushed. Gently guide them if they are having difficulty.

Use visual clues such as show them with your hand where to sit the cup so that it does not fall.

Walk down memory lane with them. That is always an excellent way to bring back special memories and make them feel better and help everyone feel relaxed.

Even if you have heard the story before, make it look like you are interested and show positive responses to their memories.

Remember what works today, may not work tomorrow.

For me, I have found that soft music and music from the fifties helps a bit for him to relax. It relaxes me at the same time.

I took a course on how art, music and dance can help someone with different forms of dementia or Alzheimer's, but the course also talked about touch therapy and how that can become an essential part of someone's day when they do not respond to other stimulation. They can still respond to touch. So allow someone to touch different fabrics and textures as this can be soothing and restful.

Massage their hands or arms as you speak to them as this also has a very soothing effect.

A Sense of humour is so critical to the health of someone. People with Alzheimer's and dementia can still have social skills and enjoy laughing with you.

Remember you are better off if you accommodate the illness and accept it for what it is. To try and control things you are probably going to be met with resistance and even anger.

Never forget there is help out there.

Cherish the good moments and be strong through the bad.

Home Safety Tips:

Some of these I have gotten from the Alzheimer's Association.

A person's abilities change as the disease progresses with Alzheimer's, Dementia and Lewy Body. Therefore it is essential that we keep the surrounding as safe as possible, including the home where they are living.

Their sense of place and time is quickly forgotten. How to get home etc., so I suggest that a bracelet with their name, address and phone number be on the bracelet so that should they become lost, this information will be with them. Hopefully, someone will see the bracelet and view this information.

A person's judgment can be altered, such as forgetting how to use appliances or turn things off. You should consider removing the knobs off the stove. Or install a gas valve or circuit breaker on the stove so a person with dementia cannot turn it on. Use appliances that have shut off features. Keep them away from sinks and other water sources.

I found that their Physical ability is drastically altered and balance becomes a real issue. Therefore it is essential to make sure that you have proper lighting throughout the home and also outside. Stairways and hallways need to have night lights and walkways outside need to have solar lights as well as motion lights.

It is also essential that floors and any surfaces inside or out where the person is walking are kept clear of debris. Remove things that someone can trip over.

Make sure that all of your safety devices are in good working order, such as fire extinguishers, smoke detectors, carbon monoxide detectors and alarm systems and any other methods you may have.

Grab bars in the washrooms are great. Put one in the shower or tub, beside the toilet and also by the sink. Grab bars will allow for safe, independent movements throughout the washroom.

Keep a list of emergency phone numbers beside a phone. Local police, fire department, hospitals and poison control helplines. You never know when you might need them in a rush.

A person can become easily confused and think that a caregiver is going to harm them. So make sure that all guns and weapons are removed from the home.

Lock up all cleaning products, detergents and bleach.

Never leave medications out in the open. Put these under lock and key in a drawer or cabinet.

Evaluate your home and also the garage and workshop. Look for hazards that can be of a danger to someone who is confused. Don't forget to check out the basement as well for things that can be a threat to them. Look for tools, chemicals and cleaning supplies that could require supervision.

Try not to make your home feel like a jail because it has become too restrictive. The house should encourage independence.

Try to keep it a social place as well. It is vital that people come and visit as it will help to keep the person with social skills and not start to withdraw.

There is clothing out there for people with Alzheimer's and Dementia:

As the disease progress, it does become an issue for the person to be able to dress. Therefore adaptive clothing may be needed, depending on the effect that the disease is having on the person.

Also, different people can have different needs. There are clothes designed to help the patient and also the caregiver looking after them.

Remember that simplicity is best. If the person can still dress or with little help, then it is best to choose clothes that have only a few buttons or choose garments with a zipper, or they pull over the head. Fewer steps mean less distress and the probability of success.

I found that in the early stage of Lewy Body and Parkinson's disease, that for John, shirts with snaps rather than buttons where a blessing. He did not have to struggle trying to do up a button.

Organize a dresser drawer, so that clothes are easily accessible. You could also organize a closet by grouping items so that it is easier to make a selection. This can be a great help to someone who is still mostly independent.

When the disease progresses, and the person now needs help, it is still the most comfortable for the caregiver to use pullover the head shirts and sweater. Even track pants can be comfortable as they have no zipper to contend with, making dressing simpler.

As the disease progresses, you will find that limited mobility, dexterity, strength and sometimes incontinence can make it challenging for people to retain their dignity.

To help someone stay warm and comfortable it is helpful to layer clothing, but remember that the person may not be able to indicate if there is a temperature problem. So always keep an eye on someone to determine if they are getting too hot or too cold.

Necessary to change their clothes regularly, as they may forget the last time they changed that shirt, etc.

As the disease progresses, the person ability to do things slows down you will have to allow for more time to dress someone. It is important not to rush them and use clothing that is easy for you to get on the person.

Always encourage personal grooming as this makes them feel better and look better.

Items that can be a big help for someone with Alzheimer's, Dementia and Lewy Body:

A clock with a large digital face that spells out the full date is a great idea. One with a non-glare display can be useful for anyone with vision problems. In case someone has a hard time to determine if it is day or night, then a clock can help tell if it is morning, afternoon or night.

Big large print calendars are an essential way to remember dates. A large wall calendar is also hard to miss and helps keep track of dates, appointments and special occasions.

Mind games are an excellent way to keep the mind active and also introduce a social aspect. Match shapes and colors. Match the dots on dominos. Playing cards like match the suits can also be fun and rewarding. People who liked Monopoly when they where young could benefit playing this game. Even a game of Grab and Go search puzzles which feature a simple layout and larger print.

Get prescriptions in blister packs at the drug store. They will do this for you. It is an excellent way of making sure that pills are taken each day.

Picture Phones. It is crucial that the person be able to stay connected with family, friends and neighbours. A memory phone can be programmed with numbers and images so that the user only has to push the person's button to call them.

An alarm system that goes off if you have also fallen this is important for anyone still living alone. The Emergency Alert bracelet if the person you are caring for wanders off.

There are many innovative products on the market today to enable those with Alzheimer's disease, dementia or other forms of memory loss to live safely, whether they are fully independent or not. These products are great for the person with any disease, but they are also a blessing for the caregiver and family member to ensure that their loved one is safe.

Exercise:

Living a Physically active lifestyle can have a significant impact on anyone with Alzheimer's, Dementia, and Lewy Body.
Benefits:

Exercise can improve the heart and blood vessels which can reduce the risk of high blood pressure and heart disease.

Helps to maintain healthy muscles and makes the joints more flexible which helps to make people more independent longer.

Decreases the risk of Osteoporosis, (a disease that affects the bones, making them weak and more likely to break.)

Helps to improve the ability to dress, clean, cook, and perform other daily activities.

Recent studies have shown that exercise may help improve memory and slow down mental decline.

Helps with improving sleep.

Exercise can help reduce the risk of falls by improving strength and balance and help to improves confidence.

Helps to improve someone's mood.

Exercise can be a good way of meeting people and reduce the feeling of isolation.

Talk to your Doctor before beginning any exercise program.

Dance and Dementia:

Relaxation should be an essential part of the day as it increases the number of endorphins in the brain which result in the sense of well being and rhythmic movements can also help you feel calmer.

Mind & Body Connection: Dance therapy helps ease problematic behaviours such as agitation which are frustrated with their changing abilities. It helps to calm down, reassuring, boosts self-confidence and self-esteem.

Motor Ability Skills: It enhances motor functioning helping with balance and coordination. It is also useful for individuals with Parkinson's as it helps to maintain motor functioning.

Communication: It allows the individual to express body language, non-verbal behaviours and also regulate emotions.

It helps to increase confidence, social and communication skills as well as improve self-esteem and overall attentiveness in individuals.

Agitation Management: Non-verbal individuals in late dementia often become agitated out of frustration and sensory overload from the inability to process environmental stimuli. Engaging them in signing and dancing, physical exercise and other structured music activities can diffuse this behaviour and redirect their attention. It stimulates memory and provides opportunities for reminiscence.

Emotional Closeness: As dementia progresses, individuals can lose the ability to share their thoughts and gestures of affection with their loved ones. However, they retain their ability to move to music until very late in the disease.

Get a Doctor's approvals before beginning any kind of exercise program including dance exercises.

How Art Therapy Enhances the Quality of Life for Dementia and Lewy Body:

It is an amazing and powerful outlet for anyone with Alzheimer's, Dementia, and Lewy Body and also for the caregivers.

Art therapy can give a person an outlet to express themselves. It can honor their lives and help to restore and build on their sense of self-worth. At the same time, it can open up an image into what and how they feel. Art therapy can be educating for a caregiver.

As someone creates art, it helps to stimulate the brain and has the power to trigger lost memories, and when the cognitive abilities decline, art is the perfect medium for non-verbal engagement.

Art uses a different part of the brain creating new paths between brain cells and wakes up dormant areas of the mind.

Some people create beautiful pieces of art for others to enjoy. They can lose themselves in the moment as they create. They can relate to others in the session, building relationships, and gain a sense of control over their environment. They discover new ways to express themselves through their art. It has been proven that many will improve their concentration and attention. The patients are often happier and more comfortable to care for after having an art therapy session.

Art therapy sessions can help someone develop a common interest with others and share in the sense of pride and accomplishment that comes from creating something unique. Creating art gives a sense of accomplishment and purpose.

If you wish to try this with someone, remember that you would never give anyone a project that would be demeaning or seem childlike.

Build conversation into the project. Give encouragement and when the person is taking a break or is finished; discuss what he or she has created or reminiscence.

Use safe materials, avoiding anything that could be toxic and avoid sharp tools.

Give plenty of time and remember the person does not have to finish. There is no right or wrong in this project. Never criticize.

There is no right way or wrong way to complete their project and let them know that you are proud of them no matter what they do.

Hang it up in your home so that others can see it as well and this will help to encourage them to keep creating and allow them to experience the feeling of empowerment that comes from making a work of art, even if it is not finished.

Drawing and painting can be used to trigger memories and express emotions. Sculpting can help to improve motor skills and dexterity. Sewing and knitting could be something that some people already know how to do, and this can allow them to create a functional piece that they can be very proud of and enjoy. Flower arrangements can be fun, colourful, and also help reduce stress. Scrapbooking can give a visual narrative and also maybe revisit their past.

Allow your loved one to experiment with these mediums to see what they enjoy doing.

Start with small projects. While you should be present to observe and help when necessary, remember that this time is for your loved one.

Art Therapy History:

I read this off the goodtherapy.org that I found interesting.

Art has been used by a means of communication, self-expression, group interaction diagnoses and conflict resolution throughout history.

We all learned in school about the carving on cave walls. Well for thousands of years many religions and cultures used carved idols as well as paintings and symbols, in the healing process.

It's believed that art therapy itself only began in the mid 20th century. The term "art therapy" was coined in 1942 by British artist Adrian Hill who discovered the healthful benefits of painting and drawing while recovering from tuberculosis since there were no actual classes to teach someone art therapy at that time than most care providers were educated in other disciplines and supervised by psychologists, psychiatrists and other mental health care professionals.

Positive results in therapy were often achieved by those facing problems such as:

Depression, stress, posttraumatic stress, anxiety, cancer, compassion fatigue, substance dependency and cognitive impairments.

Art can help people who feel out of touch with their emotions.

Some techniques used in therapy:

Sculpting, painting, drawing, carving, making pottery, making cards, using textiles and making collages.

Tactile Stimulation for Alzheimer's and Dementia

Think about it, everything around you has a texture, temperature and shape.
Every part of the body has nerves. If you get hurt, the nerves, send a message to the brain that "feels"; so tactile stimulation is brain stimulation!

A gentle massage can be a powerful way to connect with someone. You don't have to be a professional to give a massage. A touch to a hand or foot or a massage to the upper back or neck and can be relaxing and enjoyable.

You can use oil to provide lubrication to minimize friction with the skin. A scented oil can lend a whole other dimension to the massage such as aromatherapy. Lavender and Melissa oil which is a lemon balm both have many beneficial effects for people with dementia.

An excellent way to achieve textile stimulation is to take a walk in the woods or in a park if the person can do this. The bark on a tree is a wonderful textile as each tree is different. The touch and smell of a flower can bring back wonderful memories. The feel of leaves in their hands and the touch of green grass can also stimulate memories from years that have passed. Or if you're loved one is not capable of walking through the woods or park then bring the park to them. Bring a flower and a few pieces of bark.

A bit of moss that they can appreciate the feel of softness and pine cones and acorns can be an excellent stimulus.

You can start a collection of objects that can provide stimulation. These objects can be found almost anywhere. Some people with more advanced dementia may tend to put it in their mouths, so keep an eye on them, and never include bite-sized objects in the collection.

Researchers found that using textile stimulation helped to improve short-term memory and long-term memory in people diagnosed with Alzheimer's and Dementia. There was also an improvement in their moods. After six weeks these improvements partially remained.

Similar results were achieved by a group in the Netherlands that used peripheral tactile nerve stimulation meaning (massage).

Music Therapy and Dementia:

I have been doing music therapy with John now for several months. I start with soft music first thing in the mornings when he wakes up and is having breakfast. Then I turn on music from the fifties as this is when he would have been a teenager. It has helped to bring back a lot of memories of his youth.

It has also helped me feel more relaxed and grounded for the day that lies ahead.

I read in Today's Geriatric Medicine, which is news and insight for professionals in elder care; it states that people of all ages relate to music, making it a universal language. They believe that there is significant value in listening to music.

Dr Lehtonen, PhD, who is a professor of education at the University of Turku in Finland and also a clinical therapist for more than 25 years, uses music therapy to promote memory and a sense of self in the treatment of older adults with dementia.

Music can provoke many feelings, memories, and sensations. Music has a close relationship with the unconscious emotions which are activated with musical movement.

Even if the patient does not remember anything or who they are, they can still have strong emotional and meaningful feelings through music.

Music can enhance someone's life. It can empower people to emerge from the isolation that Dementia and Alzheimer's can impose on someone. Music therapy can improve the overall mental and physical wellbeing of dementia and Alzheimer's patients.
It helps to improve memory, and someone's mood can change drastically and give a sense of wellbeing and control over one's life.

Music can be a stimulate that promotes interest even when other approaches are ineffective.
Movements to the music can help promote muscle building.

Music is a great way to interact with others socially.

Music is a beautiful way of increasing levels of physical and helps improve mental emotional and social functioning. Music helps to enhance the quality of life.

Using songs in a therapy setting can help to stimulate a memory from the past. It can have a substantial effect on someone's mood and can be an engaging and emotional stimulus. You are giving a person a renewed sense of identity. Music can be an excellent way of keeping people happy.

Music and dance is a beautiful way to exercise. It's never too late to begin; even those who are very frail can still benefit from this type of exercise. It is essential that the music keeps the pace, and the number of repetitions. Music does make the activity seem more enjoyable and fun; this will also help to make it feel shorter and more pleasant.

It is crucial to obtain a physician's approval before starting any exercise program.

History of music therapy in Canada:

Music therapy began in the 1800s in an unofficial capacity in World War 1 and 11 when community musicians went to military hospitals around the country to play for veterans suffering from both physical and emotional trauma. There was such a positive response by the veterans to the music therapy that the hospital hired musicians. Soon the demand grew for music therapy worldwide.

By the middle of the 1950s there where independent music therapist working in Canada.

There was a survey done in the 1960s of music in hospitals. It was discovered that many hospitals used musical activities and many of the staff were trained in music.

Science has caught up with what music therapists have been witnessing for many decades- that music can change the way a person feels, thinks and behaves, giving positive stimulation to someone.

Children can have dimentia:

Even though we all think of the elderly with Alzheimer's and Dementia but unfortunately children and teens can get this disease.

Many kids may have dementia as a result of other rare diseases.

There are two children that I have read about that are called Addi and Cassi. They both have dementia. It is challenging to deal with dementia in children as they don't remember (or can't learn) that stairs are steep, things such as a stove can be hot; streets are dangerous due to cars.

These two children where once potty trained and knew their nursery rhymes but now they can't remember any of that as a result of their fatal genetic cholesterol condition that is destroying their brains.

Here are some conditions in children that involve dementia:

Adrenoleukodystrophy,
Alexander disease
Autism (infantile)
Batten disease
Canavan disease
Juvenile Huntington's disease
Metabolic disease
Niemann-Pick Type C
Subacute-sclerosing Panencephalitis (SSPE)
Tay-Sachs disease

More research needs to be done and more resources to be written and more educational efforts to bring attention to dementia and the young.

It's believed that infections and poisoning can lead to dementia in people of any age.

Dealing with Parkinson's Disease

Millions of people are diagnosed with Parkinson's disease worldwide. The cause of Parkinson's is presently not known, but research points to both genetic and environmental factors. Only about fifteen per cent of the cases are considered genetic forms, so the chances of getting the disease if it runs in the family are low.

Even though there is no cure, there are treatment options to help manage the symptoms. People with Parkinson's often experience different symptoms.

The main symptoms are the tremor and slow movements. There is generally stiffness of the trunk and limbs, impaired coordination and balance. There is a loss of automatic movements and changes in writing and speech. Speech may become soft, and there can be some slurring, hesitating or speaking too quickly, and writing can become very difficult.

Tremors can be more apparent on one side and usually begin in the fingers or hands even when at rest and the forefinger and thumb may rub each other in a circular movement. Walking becomes difficult with shortened steps and dragging feet. Stiff muscles can reduce the range of motion and cause severe pain. Stooped posture and balance may weaken when standing or walking.

Exercise has been proven to play a crucial role in maintaining a good quality of life for someone with Parkinson's disease. The range of motion exercises, strength training and other forms of physical activity can help a patient maintain mobility, dexterity and balance.

Even though exercise will not stop Parkinson's disease from progressing it will improve your balance, and it can prevent joint stiffening.

Always check with your Doctor before beginning any exercise program.

The type of exercise that works best for you depends on your symptoms, fitness level and overall health. Your Doctor will recommend what kinds of activities are best suited for you.

Generally, exercises that stretch the limbs through the full range of motion are encouraged.

Always warm up before starting any exercise routine and cool down at the end.

If you want to do 30 minutes, then start with 5 or 10-minute sessions and work your way up to the 30 minutes.

If you have difficulty with balance, then exercise with a grab bar or rail. If you have trouble standing or getting up, try exercising in bed rather than on the floor or mat.
Any time you begin to hurt then STOP.

Food and Dementia: info was taken from Dementia.org

A healthy well-balanced diet can make a big difference in the dementia's regression. The nutrients found in certain foods not only feed your body but also supply the brain.

Leafy Greens

Spinach, kale, Swiss chard, collard and mustard greens are all a great source of folate, or vitamin B9, which is shown to improve cognition in older adults. Folate fights depression which is (a common dementia side-effect) by contributing to serotonin levels. The vitamin E in leafy green veggies has shown to have positive effects on the brain.

Cruciferous Vegetables

Cabbage, cauliflower, broccoli, bok choy, and brussel sprouts all help to retain memory. They each contain carotenoids and folate, which lowers levels of homocysteine, an amino acid linked with cognitive impairment.

Beans

Legumes are full of folate and iron as well as magnesium and potassium. They contain choline, a B vitamin that boosts acetylcholine, a neurotransmitter critical for brain function.

Berries and Cherries

All varieties of berries contain anthocyanin, a phytochemical that protects the brain from damage caused by free radicals; inflammation and radiation. Blueberries are filled with the most antioxidants, as well as generous amounts of Vitamin C and E.

Dark Chocolate

Flavanols, the antioxidant in cocoa powder, help improve blood flow to the brain. The darker the chocolate, the better it is for you since you will be getting more flavanols and less sugar.

Fish

A study has shown that people over the age of 65 who ate fish enriched with omega-3 three times a week or more, had nearly 26 per cent lower risk of brain lesions that can cause dementia, compared to those who never eat fish. The high levels of omega-3 fatty acids keep the brain in tip-top shape

Nuts

A small handful of nuts put a ton of nutrients including omega-6 and omega-3 fatty acids, Vitamin E, foliate Vitamin B6 and magnesium. These nutrients help protect against age-related memory loss, as well as work to improve mood.

All varieties of nuts, including peanuts, cashews, hazelnuts, walnuts, almonds, and pecans, offer these benefits.

Seeds

Vitamin E found in seeds. This vitamin is associated with lower rates of age-related cognitive decline. Choline, a compound found in sunflower seeds, helps to improve brain function. The zinc present in pumpkin seeds enhances memory and cognitive function, while the tryptophan fights depression. Flaxseeds are an excellent alternative to fish since they are full of memory-boosting omega-3s.

Spices

Certain spices not only add flavour to your food but also add antioxidants and memory-boosting compounds. The mere scent of cinnamon, for instance, enhances cognitive processing. In a study, participants who consumed sage performed better on memory tests. And curry lovers can rejoice; Curcumin, the main ingredient in turmeric, has been shown to break up brain plaque and reduce inflammation that can cause memory problems.

NOTES

Life is measured in love and positive contributions and moments of grace.

Carly Fiorina

www.ingramcontent.com/pod-product-compliance
Lightning Source LLC
Chambersburg PA
CBHW071403210526
45465CB00001B/226